Life Constricted

Life Constricted

To Love, Hugs and Laughter

Gerald Green

To order additional copies of this book, contact:
Xlibris Corporation
1-888-795-4274
www.Xlibris.com
Orders@Xlibris.com
75484

CONTENTS

ACKNOWLEDGMENTS

I THANK MY wife, Monica, for saying, "Yes, you can." She continuously supports my dreams, which motivated me to take a writer's class taught by mystery writer Ms. Penny Warner in the summer of 1996. Ms. Judy Juanita reviewed my first attempt at writing chapter 1 and encouraged me to read *Life Wish* by Jill Ireland, Charles Bronson's late wife who died from breast cancer, to understand how pain and suffering helps sell books.

Monica later introduced me to Voices of Our Nations Arts (VONA) Foundation, where thanks to Professor Elmaz Abinader's skillful tutelage, my writer's voice started to emerge. Thanks to Diem Jones, the executive director of VONA, and other faculty members who heard it and recommended me for a writer's fellowship at Stanford University.

Ms. Melanie Hilario helped me reorganize my thoughts and recommended I shorten the book's first title: *Living Above the Line, A Family's Victory Over Cancer*. About thirteen months later, I came up with the title *Life Constricted*. Thanks to Ronald Taylor for his editorial review and for not changing my voice that Ms. Autumn Stephens helped hone. She's the captain of our motley crew of cancer survivors. We meet twice a month at Alta Bates Summit Hospital and participate in Cancer in Other Words writing workshop. Her ten- to twenty-minute writing exercises using unique writing prompts, like a bowl of pills, mentally propel us to exotic terrain. We write and read our stories to each other in order to continue our healing journey.

My cancer journey started in June 1995. Fortunately, I had purchased an excellent medical plan (Cadillac version) through my employer, Pacific Gas & Electric. I appreciate the plan administrator's timely approval of my tests and medical procedures. I am thankful to the numerous doctors and nurses and other hospital staff personnel, who sustained my life. I am also thankful for Monica's former employer, Development Associates, who extended her flexible work hours during our time of need.

My life was saved—everybody's life is precious and deserves excellent medical care. I am forever in debt to the aforementioned for their support and eternal encouragement. God bless those who prayed and continue to pray for me.

INTRODUCTION

"THAT'S NOT FAIR," Charles said. He was right; life isn't fair, but as parents, we must teach our children fairness and—to our boys especially—that no means no. My grandfather and my son's namesake, Mr. Charles Patillo, a generation removed from slavery and an entrepreneur from North Carolina, overcame racism and taught me fairness and self-reliance in segregated Virginia. I hope to pass on his wisdom to my son in post-civil rights America, while surviving cancer and evolving from Tinman to husband and father.

Cancer forced us to retreat from our hurried professional path, typical of two-income families in the Bay Area. We rearranged our priorities and lived life constricted to pursue its greatest opportunity—love that thrived on hugs, quality time, and laughter.

Similar to *Life Wish*, *Life Constricted* addresses a personal struggle with cancer but from a father's perspective. I have survived three bouts of cancer; however, this memoir mainly addresses the first discovery and treatment, and it includes a little of my second encounter. Similar to H. G. Wells's book *The Time Machine*, some sections propel the reader forward in time. I share this so others may benefit from reading about my reversal of misfortune, because cancer is an equal opportunity disease affecting millions of Americans annually.

I write to warn; be careful, sharp rocks ahead. Besides, life provides no guarantee. We must beam hope to generations unborn and give them a clue of the landscape. Young man, do you know your father? My eyes ask this of black teenagers at the Oakland Mentoring Center's Fatherhood program, where I volunteer on Tuesday nights. I write to communicate the collective hope that my brothers can gain knowledge of self. We must lead the charge in solving our community problems and not wait for others to rescue us from becoming singers, actors, and athletes.

I write heartfelt love songs about Monica and fatherhood at sixty. We fathers must stimulate our boys through our actions to achieve their best. I listen to Charles play his *djembe* drum, and we talk about music and rhyme and its relationship with writing. I write so he can hear my life's rhythm. I write to motivate other black men to share their stories, so we can collectively heal our community.

I wrote many funding requests for capital and maintenance projects when I was a gas engineer with Pacific Gas & Electric. Just the facts, please, no creative voice. I wrote technical manuals, and I perfected writing letters in my supervisors', managers', and vice presidents' voices. The right side of my brain was king.

Elmaz Abinader helped my writer's transformation, and I welcome you to my voice, *Life Constricted*. Caution: time shifting ahead.

PROLOGUE

KIDS IN ELEMENTARY school pushed their noses in and called me snub-nosed .38, and others laughed at me when I stammered, "Uh . . . uh . . . sqr . . . eet," for the word *street*. Schoolmates called me Gappy Hayes because of the gap between my front teeth. My immediate family called me Jerry, and other relatives called me Cousin Jerry. This youthful preteen banter lowered my self-esteem, before I started high school in Lexington Park, Maryland, where white students called me nigger.

These taunts didn't stop when I moved to San Diego in the spring of 1966, where I introduced myself as Gerald. I was late for class one day when a black high school student shouted, "Look at that nigga walking like a tinman." Some students imitated my knock-kneed walk while others called each other names like Zit-face, Monkey-man, and Foe-head. Foe-head's real name was Paul, and he had a big smile, overshadowed by his Rock of Gibraltar-sized forehead, crowned with black kinky hair combed into a pompadour. Foe-head started calling me Tin-head because I would drink more than my share of liquor when the bottle was passed around in the car en route to parties. Foe-head was drafted and died in the Vietnam War a few years after graduating from high school.

At eighteen, I could buy alcohol from most liquor stores. My college buddies and I would collect $1.39, and I would buy a gallon of cold Red Mountain vin rosé. We called ourselves the Red Mountain for lunch bunch. I was first to get a sip. I would hook my right index finger through the circular glass ring at the top of the gallon, flip it onto my forearm near my elbow, then turn it skyward and place my lips on the bottle, all in one smooth move. Those with less experience drank from cups. We jug buddies drank our wine in the college parking lot while listening to eight-track tapes, lying about women, and talking stuff about the war instead of going to class. I would discover many years later that a social club in New Orleans called the Jug Buddies drank their liquor in a rented hall after the Mardi Gras parade.

I went to Mesa Community College in San Diego to evade the draft. I partied more than I studied data processing and wrecked my white convertible returning home late one night. Many times my father had told me, "As long as you live in my house, you will obey my rules. And I don't care how late you stay out, you're going to church." I struggled getting up in time for church and felt like a hypocrite sitting in the pew with a hangover. When Dad returned from six months at sea, he sought solace on the golf course instead of spending quality time with us. His absences caused marital tension and emotionally wounded me and my brothers, pain I thought moving out would help heal. I moved to the Top-Notch Studio Apartments next to the Aztec Taco Shop, then home of the ten rolled tacos for a dollar. I was evicted after thirty days because of loud music and moved into another apartment, which became known for underage drinking, smoking weed, and partying most nights.

I relocated to the Bay Area to attend a dental technology school the summer of 1969. I carved bicuspids and molars during the day and took little white diet pills in the evening to help me flip burgers until early the next morning, when I would return home and blast my Motown-listening roommates with Jimi Hendrix. We lived within earshot of a park across the street from the Berkeley police station where electrified bands blasted deafening vibrations on Sunday; and people drank alcohol, dropped acid, and smoked weed with no fear of arrest. It was the type of activity the police wouldn't have tolerated from an all-African American crowd.

Eighteen-hour days coupled with long bus commutes didn't allow me time to socialize. I dropped out of school but kept my job flipping burgers at the Doggie Diner. I started partying more and introduced myself as Tinman because that persona wasn't afraid of rejection and was immune to those hurtful words that made Jerry and Gerald feel inadequate.

In time I attempted to rein in Tinman.

CHAPTER 1

Click Click

GROUND-UP POPCORN KERNELS oozed under my partial dentures. I tried ignoring the pain, but the gritty mess robbed the popcorn taste. I flushed it down with pink lemonade between bites until my gums screamed.

That hurts!

I don't know why I expected a different result; the same thing happened every time I ate popcorn. I quit eating, removed my partials, and wrapped them in a napkin. I took my eyes off the movie screen for a second while putting the false teeth in my pocket. Damn, I missed it. *What happened?* Everyone laughed except me. Then the joke hit me, but tongue spasms stole the humor. The cool drink didn't stop the creeping agony. Mentally, I returned to a dental visit with Dr. Curtis Perry during the spring of 1995.

He loved electronic devices and offered me special glasses to watch him work on my teeth. I declined the offer and listened to music instead. Dr. Perry told me how he had started a jazz band called Schedule II, which is the script name for state-control drugs. He played the bass guitar and had a weakness for chocolate. I, on the other hand, loved playing the phantom bass with Jimi Hendrix. Music stitched our fabric together.

Dr. Perry became a dentist, like his father. My father was a photographer in the navy. He taught me how to evaluate pictures, but I couldn't stand all the posing in front of his tripod. I hated watching him salute white men who thought my father was beneath them. I rebelled and didn't become seriously motivated to attend college until I was twenty-five. Dr. Perry went straight through college and medical school. He always seemed so optimistic, a trait the news media fail to tell about Oakland's African American males.

Dr. Perry must have gotten an A in smile class 101 at medical school because he instilled trust. My frown lines needed smile rehab; however, witnessing his was contagious. I prayed for infection.

During a routine exam, Dr. Perry touched my tongue with an instrument. "Does that hurt?" he asked.

"Yes!" I jumped. He took a deep breath.

"Oh, that doesn't look good," he said. I couldn't see his concern through my tears, and my ears buzzed. I barely heard him say "You have a lesion on your tongue."

"A lesion," I blurted. "I thought it was from biting my tongue."

"No, that's more than a tongue bite," he said before entering something in the computer next to my chair. I felt crushed, trapped between fear and anger. I had ignored the stinging sensation for days, and now uncertainty raised unanswered questions.

Dr. Perry recommended a follow-up visit with a Dr. William R. Murphy, a specialist in oral and maxillofacial surgery. Dr. Perry had used Dr. Murphy's services before. He specialized in sedating patients to pull difficult teeth, and his office was walking distance from Dr. Perry's office.

"Please stick out your tongue. Hold it," Dr. Murphy said at my first visit.

I felt childish, and the smooth jazz from the overhead speakers didn't stop my jitters. Dr. Murphy's frown showed concern.

"Now move your tongue to the left and touch your top lip," he said.

I complied; saliva filled my mouth and spilled on the bib. He instructed his nurse to place a suction tube in the corner of my mouth and then continued to probe my tongue. I did not know it at the time, but this would be the first of many examinations, where a doctor would touch my tongue with their latex-covered fingers or stick small mirrors in my mouth and tell me to say ah!

We repeated the same ritual at my next visit, just four days before my son's first birthday. After the examination, I saw signs of alarm on Dr. Murphy's face. My stomach muscles tightened, and terror replaced rational thoughts. Tingling nerves made me sweat. I scanned the room for comfort.

"Most injuries heal after fourteen days," he said. "It has been over twenty days since your last visit." He requested permission to conduct a biopsy.

"Please . . . Can you wait and observe it one more time?" I stammered. He didn't smile.

"We must act soon," he said.

I tried to imagine a dentist cutting out a portion of my tongue, but the thought of cold hard steel against my tongue ignited my fear. How could I allow a medical inquisition into my most intimate muscle, designed from birth to nurture my body and articulate thoughts from my soul? Later that week, Monica and I celebrated Charles's first birthday. Charles crawled, smiled, and laughed as he played with other children. I enjoyed watching them. His antics helped me release suppressed thoughts of those unpleasant visits to Dr. Murphy. I ate Monica's delicious spaghetti dinner. My tongue cramped with spasms, but I was determined nothing would interfere with Charles's birthday, not even my slipping partials.

One week after Charles's birthday, Monica went on a business trip to Washington DC. She returned through New Orleans to check on her mother who was recuperating from a heart attack. I called and talked about everything but never mentioned my growing anguish. The last thing she needed was more melancholy news. That night I tried to ignore the syncopated throbbing which became more frequent and intense, and over-the-counter painkillers failed. My original decision to delay the biopsy haunted me. I surrendered to pain's grip and called Dr. Murphy the next morning for an appointment. It was time for a biopsy, time to confirm what these two men of medicine believed was going on inside me.

I dropped Charles at child care and went to work, although my biopsy was scheduled for 11:00 am. And my mouth throbbed. I tried not thinking about it. Stuck in traffic, I shifted my thoughts from the biopsy to my application for graduate school. That did not help, so I turned on Bob Marley and floated on thoughts about our last vacation in Negril, Jamaica, as I inched along the highway. I arrived at work with Caribbean breezes blowing pleasant reggae melodies in my head. My pain and apprehension vanished.

All of that changed when I arrived at work. I double-checked the status of a few of my projects and felt like NASA getting ready to launch a space shuttle, "T minus two hours, twenty-two minutes, and twenty-one seconds and counting." Thoughts about 11:00 am kept my work rhythm offbeat. My phone, my neighbors' phones, all the phones rang and annoyed me. I couldn't think, my heart rate doubled, and my body ached. It was time to go. I hit a time blitz and slipped over the rolling June-dried hills through the Caldecott Tunnel into Oakland. The cold reality of my biopsy hit me, accelerating my mental countdown: *T minus twenty minutes and ten seconds*. I parked in front of Dr. Murphy's office and hummed a tune. Inside, the receptionist's smile failed to console my fear.

"Hello, Mr. Green," she said. "Please be seated. Dr. Murphy, will see you in a minute." The music in the waiting area relaxed my anxiety, and dreams of dancing with Monica flooded over me with flowing doves. Then, thoughts about the procedure cascaded; perspiration sprinkled down my beard and moistened my neck. I scanned a *Jet* magazine, not reading, just looking at headlines and pictures. My eyes darted back and forward, every now and then slowing down for juicy details.

T minus sixty long, pulsating seconds.

"Follow me," a nightingale voice sang from a petite coffee complexion. My rigid six-foot two-inch, 235-pound body stood and followed her.

"Have a seat," she said, as if I did not know the routine by now. I sat frozen and rested my wet hands on the cool leather arms of the dental chair. I forced my eyes to focus on the speakers and visualize the jazz performers, but that failed to calm me. Dr. Murphy, knowing I loathed pain, offered me a topical sedative for my gums.

"Relax your tongue," he said. He waited. It seemed like an eternity. He then eased a long needle into my gum, reloaded his elixir, and injected various nerves throughout my tongue and mouth.

"Do you feel that?" he asked. He touched the side of my tongue.

"I think so," I said. He waited a little longer, and I slipped deeper into the chair, trying not to think about his next move.

"Now . . . do you feel this?" He touched my tongue with a metal instrument.

"Yes."

Dr. Murphy gave me another injection and waited. Ten minutes passed, and I lost all sensation and feeling. I closed my eyes as Dr. Murphy began snipping at my tongue. I could hear him cutting, and my mind told me it should hurt, but I felt no pain. Dr. Murphy scooped and gouged my tongue, and my mind felt like a fish with the hook torn from its mouth, while I listened to the soothing sound of Grover Washington blowing "Winelight" on his tenor saxophone in the background. Periodically, Dr. Murphy interrupted the melody with the clicking sound of his instrument cutting and stitching as he sewed my bleeding tongue, *click, click, click, click.*

"Mr. Green, I am finished. Now, that was not all that bad, was it?" A warming sensation permeated my mouth. I swallowed blood before answering.

"No."

Dr. Murphy warned me not to eat anything until the anesthesia wore off because I could mistakenly bite my tongue and not know it. His staff provided me some gauze and a prescription for some painkillers.

"I should have the pathology report back by Wednesday," Dr. Murphy said.

It was past noon; and my breakfast of grits, two scrambled eggs with cheese, and hotly seasoned turkey sausage seemed like a distant memory. Midday hunger made gurgling noises from my stomach, but I could not eat. My tongue bled, and Dr. Murphy's warning haunted me. I decided to take the rest of the day off.

*　　*　　*

Driving toward Lake Merritt, I thought about the first time I met Monica, and that thought pushed aside my pain and hunger. Twelve years earlier, I had ridden a bus from San Francisco to the Lake Merritt area and met with members from various organizations to develop a book about the contributions of African American scientists and inventors. I had arrived early and startled the host, Monica. When she opened the door, her radiant face looked up at me.

"Hi, I'm Gerald. Isn't there a meeting here?"

I tried not to stare, but my eyes ventured beyond her face. Our eyes reunited and waltzed.

"Yes," she said, then hesitated. "I'm Monica, please come inside."

We produced a book, *Contemporary African American Scientists and Inventors 1920-Present*. As I drove past the Mormon temple, I recalled how it shared our family room view from our Laurel District home, the house that mysteriously caught fire on July 7, 1990, at 10:57 am. Monica and I survived the fire and watched many of our personal belongings burn before firefighters extinguished the flames.

We moved temporarily into a lovely marina condo in the Watergate Condominium in Emeryville while we rebuilt our home. The fire gutted our upstairs, approximately a year before the Oakland Hills fire. Like many Oakland Hills survivors, we took the opportunity to remodel. We raised the roof five feet, which essentially doubled the size of our house and added high vaulted ceilings to the family room and master bedroom. Monica added recessed lights to accent our art. I designed our master bedroom suite complete with bath and redwood deck, after a room we shared at the Russian River Jazz Festival. Perhaps this flashback was preparing me mentally for the future—to soar like the phoenix.

I stopped at Walgreens on 106th Avenue to pick up my pain prescription, before I drove past the Oakland Zoo on the way home. All the driving and the new pain prescription made me sleepy. Despite my hunger, I lapsed into a deep sleep at home. Just before I dozed off, my thoughts became preoccupied with food, especially the sweet potato pie that I had eaten on my forty-sixth birthday.

I woke up in time to get Charles.

*   *   *

Monica's airport limousine pulled in front of the house shortly after Charles and I returned home. She shimmered with excitement upon seeing us. I gave Monica a passionate big, hard, long hug; but I felt uncomfortable giving her a warm, wet kiss. The physical and emotional pain of the stitches in my tongue stopped me. Instead, I gave her a short peck on the cheek.

Monica picked up Charles and lowered her free arm to hug my waist, then up to my shoulders. I did the same as we stood in the middle of the living room in front of the cold flagstone fireplace. Monica whispered, "I love you, darling."

"I love you" flowed from her lips with ease. She always ended her calls to her mother, brother, and sister with "I love you." I rarely said, "I love you," when ending telephone conversations with my mother, brothers, and sisters. We said good-bye. Monica's and Charles's warmth enveloped me, and I said, "I love you too," as I gently squeezed them. Charles twisted, squirmed, and pulled at my beard, ending the family group hug.

Later, when Monica and I were in bed, I attempted pillow talk; but thoughts about my biopsy squashed romantic foreplay.

"How was your trip, baby?" I asked. Monica adjusted her arms to hug my pillow.

"The time in Washington dragged on and on with each meeting. I'm glad I visited Momma on my return trip," she said. I tried to ignore her body language.

"How was she?" I asked. Monica sensed my indifference and changed her tone.

"Her recovery is running slightly ahead of schedule, and she looks great," she said and paused.

"Momma asked about you and Charles."

"She did," I said, fidgeting with the sheet. Monica released her hug on my pillow and pushed away.

"How was your day?" she asked.

My voice cracked and I stammered. "Well, today was really rough."

She looked at me for a clue.

"I had a biopsy on my tongue," I said, staring blankly at a picture on the wall. Her body flinched; her eyes peered through me.

"Oh, Gerald!" she said. Silence separated us.

"The results will be available on Friday." Neither of us talked. Instead, we hugged. Monica fell asleep. My mind raced. Memories from 1993 of completing the course A Model Approach to Partnerships and Parenting at the Black Adoption Placement and Research Center washed over me. I recalled how satisfied and fulfilled I felt a year later after Charles entered our lives. Pleasant thoughts about Charles and Monica coupled with her warm embrace relaxed my apprehension, and then sleep came.

Wednesday, Dr. Murphy called me at work. He asked, "Have you ever smoked? How long did you smoke? Do you drink? What and how much?"

I suppressed Tinman's escapades and answered his questions.

"I recommend you bring your loved one to the appointment," Dr. Murphy said.

I suspected a problem, but forced my attention on work, shutting out his words like I had done Monica; and I didn't tell her about his tone. I felt threatened and suspected bad news, but thoughtlessly didn't prepare her mentally for our doctor visit.

CHAPTER 2

The Second Line

FRIDAY, JUNE 30, 1995, started for us with a 7:30 am one-year medical examination appointment for Charles with Dr. Gary Bean, a childhood friend of Dr. Perry. Dr. Bean's smile transmitted warmth and confidence, and he too must have received an A in smile class. He had played in Schedule II, Dr. Perry's band, and his office and his examination rooms were full of beautiful black-and-white pictures of jazz performers. He had captured their sweat, grunts, and strained smiles in perfect harmony with their lyrics. I appreciated his craftsmanship. It reminded me of those 1950s pictures taken by my dad.

Charles weighed nineteen pounds, two ounces, which placed him below the fifth percentile on the growth curve. Charles received a shot and a TB skin test as part of his examination. His piercing cries lowered to a whimpering murmur shortly after Dr. Bean placed a San Francisco 49er Band-Aid on his arm. I wished the same remedy would work for me. Seeing Charles's little body in pain reminded me of my previous visits to Dr. Murphy. After Charles's appointment, Monica and I rushed Charles to child care before my 9:00 AM appointment with Dr. Murphy.

"Mr. and Mrs. Green, the doctor will see you now," the receptionist said. Monica smiled, and I stolidly stood, helped her up. We entered the office. I examined floor tiles. She looked at the ceiling.

"Good morning, Mr. and Mrs. Green, please be seated," Dr. Murphy said. He was a slight man with a polite smile, not like some of those champion Wal-Mart greeters. We sat in front of his desk flanked by family pictures of fishing trips and other vacations. Seeing those pictures brought back glum memories of Dad and me baking in the sun, fishing from a rowboat—we seldom caught anything. I felt trapped and hid suspicion of bad news from Monica. She relaxed in her chair, and we engaged Dr. Murphy in conversation. Our eyes were drawn to a vanilla folder. He picked it up from a pile, and the room became quiet.

"Mr. Green, I have your pathology report," he said. Our nervous energy warmed the room. We held hands and peered at the messenger.

"Mr. Green, I'm sorry to tell you, but your report showed malignant cells. You have squamous cell carcinoma, cancer of the tongue."

Our hands broke apart. I choked, then gasped for air, and moisture escaped my mouth. I looked at Monica crying and wanted to say something comforting but sat speechless. Dr. Murphy's words—*cancer of the tongue*—continued to reverberate. Monica's face pleaded for help, and I did nothing. Her tears spilled to the floor, and her gut-wrenching sobs echoed in my ears. I wanted to hold her tight but didn't and retreated to my youthful safe harbor; and when I opened my eyes, I saw strained, uncomforting lines on Dr. Murphy's face.

"I will leave you two alone for a few minutes," he said.

He stood and pointed to the restroom. Monica didn't see my quivering hand. She ran into the restroom. I felt lost. The walls swallowed me. Cancer digested my energy. My soul sang, *Gerald, you must live, live for your son, live for your wife, live for yourself, just live!* I licked my lips and sang quietly to myself until Monica returned.

"Baby, don't cry, we'll make it through this," I said. We hugged. Her crying slowed, but she still hadn't said a word. Silence heightened my anxieties, and my fears grew worse.

"Tongue cancer is generally treated by partial tongue removal," Dr. Murphy said. "Typically 50 percent if the cancer is detected early." His voice grew mute, and so did my brain. Then uncontrollable thoughts returned and violated my spirit.

What's going to happen to us? I thought.

"Do you know of other treatments?" I asked.

"No," he answered.

My untarnished optimism pushed his answer aside. Monica seemed to have hung on every word, and she continued to struggle with her tears.

"Dr. Murphy, we have another appointment," I said.

"Where should I send the pathology report?" Dr. Murphy asked. I gave him my personal physician's telephone number.

Monica and I left speechless and didn't talk much en route to Saint Mary's College where I dropped off my application for the executive MBA program. My personal physician, Dr. Geoffrey Watson, thought my efforts were misguided. But I had watched my coworkers get MBAs and promotions. I wanted the same opportunity to climb the middle management ladder. On the way home, I chose the serene back road filled with steep curves circling up and down the peaceful watershed landscape. I accelerated through them. I felt my dreams helplessly slip away. Cancer became my copilot.

Monica had grown up driving in the Rocky Mountains, but now heights made her anxious. She had complained before about my driving on trips across elevated bridges, over rolling hills, and up steep inclines. She gripped her seat through each curve. I sought mental release by driving fast over the roller coaster—like road, until I heard trembling in her voice.

"Baby, please slow down," she said. I eased my foot off the accelerator, and the trees no longer flickered by.

"Thanks, Gerald," she said, twisting in her seat, holding on to the armrest. I felt ashamed.

*　　*　　*

Cancer's unknown fate threatened our wedding vows. I slipped into a world dependent on Monica's strength, yet her spirit cried sad songs. She made numerous calls to her sister Yvonne in Denver for support and relied on her twin cousins to soothe her with refrains of

> O coz, you're not alone
> Just lean on us
> Just lean on us.

Barbara, one of the twins, rejuvenated Monica when I was hospitalized, calming her nights alone with Charles, with a simple call.

"Hi, coz, how you doing?"

"Oh, Barbara, it's been a rough night."

Barbara's father, Emile, was one of Monica's father's older brothers. Emile settled in Richmond, California. He had fought next to artillery fire in World War II and, as a result, lost most of his hearing. He had inherited entrepreneurial grace from his Caribbean ancestors. As a boy, he honed his craft by buying vegetables on the Mississippi River and selling them in uptown New Orleans. Emile was retired from selling real estate and fighting prostate cancer when I introduced him to my mother, Rotelia, the year we were married. Emile often served fried fish and conducted adult Sunday-school class at home.

"Emile, your fried fish is almost as good as mine," Rotelia said between bites.

"He can't hear you," I answered. Emile's hearing aid buzzed loudly. Mother licked her lips and took another piece of fish, and everyone shouted. Mother and I shared thin lips and long narrow fingers. Her cousins would take one look at me and say, "That's Rotelia's boy."

Emile's twin daughters, Barbara and Beverly, shared his love for food and conversation. Barbara, Ms. Diva, loved pink, a key color to accessorizing her outfits. She enjoyed cooking while Beverly preferred simple hairstyles and enjoyed listening to others. Beverly's favorite color is purple, and she is known as Ms. Reserved. However, they both loved to talk. When Emile joined his ancestors in 1996, everyone joked that the twins spoke loudly in case God ran out of batteries.

Barbara married Nelson Scott after he saw a picture of Beverly in the local newspaper. He read about Beverly's volunteer service, decided to attend a local dance in her honor, and threw out his lines, "Hi, Beverly, you're looking good. Would you like to dance?" Unknown to him, he was talking to Ms. Diva.

"Yes, darling," she said, smiling like a Cheshire cat.

Twenty-five years later, Monica and I helped Nelson and Barbara renew their wedding vows, the Sunday before I entered Summit Hospital for cancer treatment. Barbara and Beverly had one daughter each, who grew up like sisters, just like Monica and the twins, who helped her release emotional trauma with

> O coz, you're not alone
> Just lean on us
> Just lean on us.

Their simple refrain helped save Monica from venturing down divergent paths laced with false hope, when Charles and I demanded more from her than what she could give alone. She heard, "You're not alone, just lean on us."

*　　*　　*

Monica's brother Jimmy added his pulsating melodic rhythms to the twins' refrain. His pop's elementary schoolmates affectionately called themselves the 39ers because they graduated from New Orleans's McDonogh 35 High School in 1939. He started playing drums in elementary school, and years later, created the Jimmy Scott Coast-to-Coast Orchestra, which featured the voice of California and the Nebraska Wizard on the sax (creator of "Pay Day Jump," "Be Good to Me," and "Cold Blooded Woman"). Most of his classmates grew up playing music in the New Orleans jazz tradition. He taught his children to drum, but only Jimmy perfected the craft. Now, the 39ers play in heaven and talk about the good old days.

Monica's father served four years in a navy band in Washington State during the 1940s before he relocated his family to Richmond, California, near his brothers Arthur and Emile. Arthur had graduated from Xavier University in New Orleans with a degree in pharmacy, but no one would hire a Negro pharmacist in 1950s Vallejo, California. All three brothers were politically active in the NAACP, and when Monica was a year old, her father's leadership role attracted FBI attention during Senator Joe McCarthy's quest to rid America of communists. The NAACP Legal Defense Fund's attorney, Thurgood Marshall, defended him in court. Their oldest child, Jimmy, suffered from extreme eczema and asthma. Doctors told them that Colorado or Arizona were the best locations for his health. Mr. Scott was a civil servant and relocated to Denver to work for the federal government.

Mr. Scott learned New Orleans—style music, which was influenced by African slaves' drumbeats and guttural chants from the Crescent City's past—the blue note tones. He tapped those rhythms as he sauntered and danced to the Calvin Keys Trio at our wedding reception in the fall of 1991. He had that big father-of-the-bride smile, waving his white table napkin above his head in traditional New Orleans steps called the second line: a partying dance step congregations did during burial rituals in New Orleans. The trio recognized his gesture and started playing "When the Saints Go Marching In." Monica's patron saint was Saint Monica, the patient, enduring mother of Saint Augustine. Her spirit lived in Monica's heart. Mrs. Scott joined her husband, and everyone danced the second line around tables in La Casa de la Vista, located on Treasure Island in the middle of the San Francisco Bay.

*　　*　　*

We had just finished lunch and retreated to the patio near the pool.

"I'm scared. I don't know what's going to happen," I said.

"Yes, I know," she said, caressing my fingers. "We'll get through this together."

I repeatedly moved my left thumb across her fingers. "I've never felt this way before," I said, gently moving my fingertip up and down a vein in Monica's arm, warming her into a high school—girl giggle.

"Stop, you're making me—" she said. Her laughter stopped. "We're going to make it." I know Monica believed that more than I. She spoke with conviction provided by her faith in God.

"I don't know which is worse, fear or uncertainty," I said. "I find myself thinking about death, but I don't want to."

"Then don't," she said with a fading smile. She held my hand and comforted me.

"But I can't control my thoughts," I said.

"I know, baby. Don't worry. Things will get better, things will get better," she said, in an attempt to spare my suffering. She couldn't relieve me of my fear and uncertainty that chipped away my optimism and stole my self-control—a throwback to Tinman. I retreated inward and became more dependent on Monica. Her foundation was built on Saint Ignatius Loyola Church in Denver, where she attended from second grade through college. Her family had maintained lifelong relationships with many friends and parishioners.

I, on the other hand, attended six different elementary schools, three different middle schools, and two high schools. I started high school in Great Mills, Maryland, six years after the Little Rock Nine entered Central High School in Little Rock, Arkansas. I was one of five black students among approximately five hundred white students, and they called me nigger and physically harassed me every day without relief.

*   *   *

While waiting for Monica and Charles to return home, I smoked some catfish and prepared a pasta, broccoli, and cheese dish. I enjoyed cooking; however, increased tongue pain decreased my desire to cook and eat.

Monica normally called when she was delayed. I started to worry when they hadn't returned by 7:30 pm. She often visited her brother, but I didn't think to call him. I was relieved when I heard the garage door open.

"I was worried about you guys. I didn't know if something had happen," I said. "Boy! I'm glad you guys are home." Monica smiled and placed some packages on the countertop. "Is this Chinese food?" I asked.

"Yes, I stopped at your favorite place," she said. "Gerald! You cooked!"

A throbbing pain rushed from my tongue under my upper and lower partials.

"Monica, my mouth hurts. My partials are slipping, and it hurts when I talk."

"Anything I can do?" she asked.

"No," I snapped unintentionally. I retreated to the bedroom, took some pain medication, and went to bed, an unfortunate pattern that intensified and pushed me away from Monica and Charles. This time I fell asleep without turning and twisting. Sleep was a new convenience; it came swiftly and stole my fears, uncertainties, and pain. I embraced its temporary relief without understanding my dependency. I spiraled inward, tucking my emotions in between my pains. I didn't think of sleep as an escape, but as time passed, I increasingly chose it over involvement. It became my silent weapon of choice and allowed me to suppress my feelings, which made them more difficult to share, locking Monica out.

CHAPTER 3

Wake Up

MY MOTHER WAS born in Norfolk, Virginia, to Charlie and Cornelia Patillo. Her parents migrated to Norfolk, Virginia, from Norlina, North Carolina, and raised five daughters. She was the youngest and loved returning to her grandfather's two-story white farmhouse surrounded by green crops and red soil. My mother's grandparents and five other families, shackled without money, once worshiped in an open-air sanctuary, a bush arbor, where they sang sweet praise to God with birds singing in the background. In 1879, they purchased land from Mr. John T. Hagood for $8 and built Chapel on the Hill Baptist Church. The founding families instituted homecoming on the third Sunday in July, and over time, the small church grew. Many families that had migrated away returned to their agrarian roots and made large annual donations to support church projects at homecoming. As a young boy, I would sit still on pews in sweltering heat next to my great-aunts fanning their perspiration-dotted faces. Watching their arms move back and forth reminded me of times when they whipped sweet potatoes into smooth pie fillings. I listened to the choir and preacher, rocking my head in cadence with the spirit, until time to feast on fried chicken, smoked ham, fresh greens, rice and gravy, and of course, sweet homemade pies with cake on the side.

In the early '50s, Mother and I lived with her parents when Dad was out to sea. On many Sundays, Grandmother placed fresh-made dough on top of the refrigerator. After church, my cousins and I sat on the front porch watching neighbors parade up and down Workwood Road, as the rising dough's yeasty aroma teased the air all day, before oven-baked rolls and hot butter melted in hungry mouths later at the dinner table.

My grandparents shepherded me through the intricacies of 1950s segregated Southern society. They watched over my youthful play within the boundaries of Chesapeake Gardens, one of Norfolk's colored communities. They lived with hope by day, and at night they filled their lungs with sentinel spirits from Norlina's red clay and prayed for guidance and protection the next day.

I helped Granddaddy clean white people's churches.

"Does we pray to the same God?" I asked. Charlie's majestic black face smiled.

"Yes." And he taught me how to line up chairs in rows. He paid me a couple of quarters, unlike Dad years later, who did not pay anything when he would drop me off on hot, humid Maryland days with a jug of water and a hoe. Dad left me to clear weeds from black dirt while he went to play golf. Flies and gnats chewed on my backside as I bent over and hoed until raw blisters broke open and oozed pus. I returned every day until the weeds were gone and the soil planted.

Charlie returned to the red-clay plot at the Chapel on the Hill after he completed his worldly mission on September 17, 1964. His spirit helps me navigate life's choices and whispers ancestral secrets that motivate me spiritually in time of need.

*   *   *

I thought I heard a familiar voice. "Momma, how are you doing?" Monica said. She had called her for emotional support, which I wanted to provide but couldn't. She fell asleep after talking to her mother. I envied her peace of mind. I woke up distressed knowing a fresh day of agony awaited me, and I felt emotionally trapped. I looked at her taut black eyelashes above her heavenly smile, and I said a silent prayer for our son.

Oh, God, please help me through this crisis. Charles needs me. Give me time in his early years of life to nurture his soul with love and prevent self-hatred. God, let me extend my hand to him, as my grandfather did when I was a little boy in need of guidance, during my parents' temporary separation. Please allow me time with Monica to help Charles through his rites of passage and introduce him to African ritual and Kwanzaa celebrations so he may become a positive contributor and not dream of ways to escape responsibilities. Please make me whole, Lord, and allow me the privilege of growing older and wiser so I may share fatherhood life experiences with my loves, Monica and Charles.

Sunrays reflected off the beige backyard fence onto the overgrown grass and into our bedroom. I watched her eyelids separate and her cinnamon crimson lips expose her morning smile.

"Good morning, baby, did you sleep well?" I asked.

"Yes, darling," she said, moving closer to me. "I talked to Momma last night. She sounded great," Monica said.

"I'm happy . . . for you," I said. Her radiance absorbed my frowns.

"Momma asked about you and Charles."

I turned toward the sliding glass door and stared at clinging greenish mold patterns on the sunlit fence. Silence chilled the air. I became restless and turned again.

"Did you tell your mother I had cancer?" I asked.

"Yes," she replied, looking surprised I even asked the question.

"You did," I said, messing with the sheet.

"Momma sends you her love and prayers," she said.

"I don't want you telling everybody I have cancer," I said, with hands on my chest gripping the sheet between my fingers. Monica threw back the sheet on her side of the bed, got out, and looked down at me.

"I'm not telling everybody, Gerald . . . just my family," she said in a firm voice.

I looked at her nudity and stuttered, "I know, baby. That's what scares me."

*   *   *

Monday, I attempted to identify predecessors and successors scheduling sequences on my warehouse construction project but froze. Hearing Dr. Murphy's words about removing half of my tongue made me cry. I felt ashamed that I couldn't control my emotions, and I sent an e-mail to my supervisor:

> I write this memo to you with sadness and a strong sense of uncertainty. I found out on Friday, June 30, 1995, that I require major surgery. I will know more details later this week. I thought I could work today, but found that the uncertainty of the potential procedures precludes me from concentrating on fleet and project management issues today. I will call you on Wednesday.

Afterward, I wanted to run and hide, like Charles, when he would sneak Monica's glasses under the table and play with them. I couldn't think of a place to hide. Besides, how could I hide from myself? I mentally collapsed at my computer after sending the e-mail. I gathered up my belongings, logged out of my computer, and fled the building without making any eye contact. I didn't want coworkers seeing me distraught.

*　　*　　*

"Wake up, Mr. Green," Dr. Murphy said. He was sitting on a stool next to a tray of sharp instruments.

"How are you doing?" I stammered. His parental smile reminded me of my grandfather.

"Did you rest well, son?" he asked. His question returned me to my safe harbor, Norfolk, where I was called Jerry.

I rubbed my face and said, "Yes." He grabbed a needle and gave me a couple injections, then left the room. I could feel the chemicals tingling in my tongue and cheek.

"OK, open wide," he said when he returned. I complied, and he pricked me with an instrument.

"Did you feel that?" he asked.

"No," I nervously answered. Then he removed my stitches.

I left his office with a sore tongue, apprehensive about my next appointment. I drove a few blocks to Dr. Watson's office with my mouth numb with drugs. I spoke awkwardly to the receptionist and sat away from other patients to avoid idle talk. My head jerked a couple of times, rolled back, and rested on the wall before I fell asleep and recalled my first visit. I was his father's patient in the late '70s until 1985 when he decided to downsize his patient load and referred me to his son, who had just completed his residency. His father was one of three African American physicians who founded the Arlington Medical Group in 1956 in North Oakland and provided the predominantly African American community excellent medical services for over thirty years. He grew up in Norfolk, Virginia, and graduated, as my mother and her sisters did, from segregated Booker T. Washington High School.

A decade my junior, Dr. Geoffrey Watson inherited his father's good looks, taste for expensive shirts, and bedside manner. He often wore alligator shoes and fine-tailored wool suits. He set his patients at ease with a warm, sincere smile and handshake. His comforting eye contact softened the blow of unpleasant news.

My head snapped forward. I awoke and asked a man sitting next to me, "Did they call Gerald Green?" He ignored my question. I looked around the room for a nod. No one responded. I became irritated and tried to think about questions for Dr. Watson, but I couldn't concentrate.

A woman with custom-painted fingernails and stylish, pressed black hair said, "Gerald Green, come with me, please." I gasped and followed her. "Please step on the scale," she instructed me, once we were in the examination room. I pulled off my size 12 Tony Lama cowboy boots and stood on the scale.

"What are you doing?" she asked.

"I don't want my boots adding extra pounds," I said. She rolled her eyes and slid the counterbalance weight over to 230 pounds. She asked me to sit on the examining table, next to the blood pressure machine. She squeezed on the ball to increase tension in my arm.

"Your blood pressure is 130 over 80," she said. I was relieved to hear it wasn't elevated. Dr. Watson had recommended weight loss, stress reduction, and medication for my high blood pressure. I succeeded in short-term weight loss, only to gain it back plus more, which sometimes required a change in medication. She took my pulse.

"What is the nature of your visit?" she asked. I rubbed my hands together, looked at the floor.

"I'm here because I was diagnosed with cancer," I said with an aching tongue. She wrote in my chart.

"Dr. Watson will see you shortly," she said.

I knew "shortly" meant at least another twenty minutes. Waiting for Dr. Watson's service became routine and challenged my patience; however, I learned that his lack of punctuality wasn't a good litmus test for determining his quality of services. Through my ten-year-plus relationship with him, I have learned to value his diagnoses and good judgment. I appreciated his undivided attention during my visits, and I respected him for providing the same level of service to other patients. I learned over time not to get upset about waiting.

I was pleasantly surprised when he entered the room only five minutes after the nurse had left. He flashed a big smile, wearing his typical stylish pin-striped wool pants and custom-made shirt with cuff links.

"Good afternoon, Gerald," he said. "How are you doing?" His upbeat tempo comforted me, and the numbness in my mouth had subsided. I felt exposed.

"This hasn't been a good week," I said. "You know I was diagnosed with tongue cancer."

"I was surprised when Dr. Murphy called me," he said. His mannerisms seemed encouraging. "When I was a medical student at Vanderbilt, my librarian friend at Fisk rejected conventional treatment," Dr. Watson said. His tone scared me.

"What happened?" I asked. He looked at me with a straight face.

"She died," Dr. Watson said. "But cancer is curable when detected early and given the proper treatment. Gerald, have you experienced any pain?"

"Yeah, at Dr. Murphy's office earlier today," I answered. He looked at me with growing concern.

"No, I mean, have you experienced severe pain before your visit with him?"

"At times," I mumbled.

"What did you say?"

"Sometimes," I said in a firmer voice.

"OK." He paused to write in my file. "I see you once smoked."

"Yeah, I quit over twenty years ago. Do you think smoking was the cause?"

"It's possible," he said. I didn't share Tinman's dope-smoking legacy.

"Were you exposed to toxic chemicals?" he asked.

"I use to pump leaded gasoline in the '70s and use to work with paint ingredients when I attended college."

"It's hard to tell if smoking, in combination with chemical exposure and drinking, made you more susceptible to cancer," he said. "Some people are predisposed to certain types of cancers." I became fixated; it's my fault.

"OK, let's have a look, open. Say ah." He firmly pressed his hands on my upper and lower neck. "Does this hurt?"

"No," I said.

"OK. I didn't feel any abnormality or swelling in your lymph nodes," he said. "That's a good sign." I looked at him with lost-puppy-dog eyes.

"Why?" I asked.

"It means we caught the tumor before it metastasized," he said. I felt happy but confused.

"I don't understand," I said.

"It means that the tumor hasn't spread to your lymph node glands, the body's first line of defense against cancer," he said. Light flickered off his gold cuff link—finally some good news—we didn't do a high-five celebration, but he could tell my spirits were lifted. He wrote on a pad, looked up some information in a book he kept in a drawer, and handed me a referral.

"Gerald, call this number and make an appointment for an x-ray and a MRI."

"What's a MRI?" I asked.

"MRI stands for magnetic resonance imaging. It uses magnetic waves to make images of the inside of your body," he said.

"I understand magnetism."

"I forgot you're a mechanical engineer," he said. I twisted my wedding band on my finger to work up some courage.

"Doctor, I need your help on a personal issue," I said.

"What can I do?" he asked.

"Since I have been diagnosed with cancer, I don't want to share it with anyone . . . other than Monica," I stammered.

"That sounds normal," he said.

"But, I've asked her not to tell anyone."

"For how long?" he asked. My eyes raced around the windowless room, searching for support.

"I don't know. It's selfish, but that's how I feel," I said. "What do you think?"

"Gerald, everyone is different," he said. Beads of sweat rolled down my neck.

"What do you think about my way?"

"I don't think one way is right or the other wrong," he said. "By not telling anyone, you're refusing emotional support." I made partial eye contact, and my tongue started to throb.

"You're right," I said. We shared a smile before a nurse opened the door to remind him of the time. Dr. Watson looked at his watch. I felt selfish, keeping him so long.

"What's next?" I asked. He handed me a slip of paper.

"OK. Call Dr. Rice, he'll review your biopsy report," he said. "Gerald, please call anytime." Dr. Watson stood, signaling that my session was over.

"Gerald, the key is early detection and comprehensive treatment like surgery, radiation, or chemotherapy," he said and walked toward the door.

"What's considered successful?" I asked.

"Cure rates start as high as 90 percent and decrease depending on factors like early or late detection, localized versus metastasized," he said. I felt numb.

"And 'cure' means being cancer free for five years," Dr. Watson said. I didn't know what to think, but at that instant, five years seemed like an eternity.

"What happens after five years?" I asked. He had opened the door.

"Statistically, people that survive five years tend to live the remainder of their life cancer free."

"What kind of treatment did your librarian friend select?" I asked.

"It was a form of holistic treatment," he said. My eyes widened.

"I'm not opposed to holistic treatment, but I don't recommend that you select it instead of proven conventional practices," he said. I followed him out the door.

"You may find some holistic treatments coupled with spiritual meditation beneficial," he said.

"Thanks, Dr. Watson . . . you know, I don't understand how cancer works."

He turned around and smiled.

"Dr. Rice can help you with that after he reviews your x-rays and MRI," he said. I still wanted his attention.

"Do you think it's possible for me to attend graduate school in October?" I asked.

"I think planning to attend graduate school in the fall is overly optimistic," he said.

"I understand. First things first," I said. "I've found staying focused on long-term goals helps me visualize a healthy future." I followed him to the nurse's station.

"I think your visualization technique is an excellent aid to recovery," he said. "You should try relaxing and thinking about the good white blood cells fighting off the cancerous cells." I shook his hand. Dr. Watson took a file from the nurse.

"OK, Gerald, see you next week. Say hello to Monica for me."

CHAPTER 4

Flight Time

IN THE 1950S, Dad spent many hours posing us in front of his slow-shuttering black-and-white camera. He would position us in front of bright lights bouncing off white sheets, and he tirelessly rearranged us in front of his tripod, forever freezing our images on film in Washington DC projects we shared with other poor families. Some were Eastern Europeans just learning how to say nigger.

We moved to Anacostia, where I climbed the tallest tree near my house and sang at the top of my voice to planes that landed at Bolling Air Force Base. In 1959, I was in the fifth grade, and that spring we moved to de facto-segregated San Diego. My brothers and I slid on the backseat of a '59 four-door Ford sedan across apartheid America and peed into a bottle because most businesses denied us basic services. Dad couldn't tell Mother we were moving to San Diego because the navy wanted him to take pictures of nuclear bombs exploding over Pacific atolls, details we learned a half-life later. We moved into temporary housing that looked like a half-can. The furnished Quonset hut was located near the Thirty-second Street navy base.

I continued my Washington DC roaming privileges in San Diego. I was returning from the movies one afternoon, and three brown-skin boys called me nigger in a foreign accent, and I ran for my life.

Shortly after our arrival, we moved to a poor community of single-story flat-roof reclaimed World War II—era houses adjacent to the San Diego River levee, a dry, putrid cesspool riverbed consisting of rodents and weeds. Prepubescent boys and I explored the streams of earthen rot with scores of seagulls that circled above the levee and Frontier Elementary School yard, where their droppings splattered students eating lunch.

My sixth-grade teacher, Mr. Robert L. Matthews, told my mother that I didn't read at grade level and I didn't spell *Gerald* correctly all the time. He recommended I read the newspaper aloud to her to improve my reading and comprehension skills. The following year, I memorized the Nicene Creed and other prayers that helped me graduate third in my confirmation class from Saint Paul Episcopal Church. I completed the seventh grade on the honor roll. We moved a third time, into a partially furnished navy apartment on the opposite side of town.

Mother had a baby girl and named her LeAnn, after one of my sixth-grade classmates that she thought looked pretty. LeAnn was born February 2, 1962, nineteen days before I turned thirteen. I learned to stick myself instead of her when changing her diapers, a skill Mother's navy-wife friends noticed and paid me fifty cents per hour to babysit their red-bottomed babies. A talent I took to Lexington Park, Maryland, in the spring of 1963. The white folks there weren't friendly, and I felt isolated. I developed a passion for swimming and often swam laps in the pool at the Patuxent River Naval Air Station. All through school, it seemed as though we moved every third spring, and like clockwork, we returned to San Diego in the spring of 1966.

* * *

I met Ron Hayes the summer of '67 after I had graduated from high school. We moved to the Pacific Beach section of town, where Ron's white high school football teammates had called him Purple Haze with affection, after Jimi Hendrix's popular song "Purple Haze." He misunderstood because he didn't listen to Hendrix and thought they were insulting him by calling him purple black. Ron thrived on running over his opponents on the field, and at six feet two inches, his solid muscles made other jocks jealous; however, he had a kind, gentle soul and never cursed.

Our friendship grew over the years, and he told me that he had planned to move to Oakland and share an apartment with his older cousin Greg, a Vietnam vet and political science student. I told him my plans to go to school in the Bay Area, and he said I could temporarily stay with him and Greg. I met Greg when he drove his 1963 dark green Austin Healey to San Diego to pick up Ron on their way to Mexico.

"Say, Tinman, I want you to meet my cousin Greg," Ron said. I nodded.

"Greg, this is Tinman." Greg turned his head from his car and looked up through his metal-rim glasses.

"Say, brother, I'll charge you $5 to wash my car," Greg said.

"You'll charge me $5 to wash your car!" I shouted. Ron's smile went south.

"Ah man, ignore him. He's joking," Ron said.

"Ron, your cousin is weird," I said. Greg pulled his glasses forward on his nose and stroked his goatee.

"You brothers need to loosen up. I was just messing with ya," Greg said. I looked down at his short, stout body.

"Yeah, OK, man," I said.

I watched Ron get into the passenger's side of the sports car, and Greg hopped into the driver's seat. They drove to Mexico, where rocky roads south of Ensenada cracked the oil pan. Later that evening, Ron called me for a ride back to San Diego. I charged them $5 each. At the time, gas was just twenty-five cents a gallon. Greg fixed his car and returned to Oakland. Greg's brother had graduated from Career Academy School of Radio Broadcasting, and his endorsement of Career Academy convinced me that I had made the right decision to relocate, although he never attended Career Academy School of Dental Technology. I felt good about my decision.

Mother and I visited Career Academy School of Dental Technology in Los Angles in 1968. I still remember the day when she squeezed my arm until tears spilled from her eyes.

"Jer . . . Jerr . . . Jerrry, what's it doing now?" she stammered.

The jet engines roared, and the plane sped down the overcast runway.

"It's taking off, Mother," I said.

She squeezed my arm even harder. The plane made a thump-thump sound, and its wheels lifted from the ground. The force pushed us deep into our seats. She held on with her eyes closed tight.

"Mother, you can open your eyes," I said looking at the ground fade into the Pacific Ocean.

"Is it finished?" she asked. Her eyes were still closed.

"Yes, we're in the air," I said, greeting her opened eyes in search of comfort with a smile. The plane hit what seemed like a dead spot, and it stopped vibrating. The engine noise went silent.

"Jerry, it stopped flying!" Mother stammered. She looked out her window at the motionless air.

"Jerry, we're not moving!"

"Mother, look down," I said. She took a couple deep breaths and saw the plane's shadow dance atop the clouds as it zipped north up the California coast. Calm returned to her voice.

"Oh, I see, Jerry," she sighed and relaxed in her seat a little.

"Jerry, I never thought signing that paper for you meant I would take my first plane ride."

"Neither did I, Mother," I said. Her breathing relaxed a little. The plane finished its climb, and the Fasten Seat Belt and No Smoking lights went out. Mother's trembling hand reached into her purse and pulled out her lighter and a pack of Raleighs. She turned the pack upside down, and a cigarette fell into her shaking hand. She managed to put it between her lips, lit it, and took a deep puff. Other passengers did the same, and the back of the Pacific Southwest Airlines plane filled up with smoke. Shortly after some passengers finished their cigarettes and drinks, the brief flight from San Diego to Los Angeles was over.

I returned from Los Angeles to my production control job at the naval air station, where my unit managed repairs and overhauls on airplanes from aircraft carriers deployed in Vietnam. I commuted to work on a ferry called the nickel snatcher across the San Diego Bay to North Island and then caught a moving van designed to carry people, called a cattle car. I was often late and worked ten-hour days and every other Saturday.

My paychecks were packed with overtime pay; however, I paid only $30 a month for a furnished room complete with a three-piece sectional sofa, a butterfly-shaped love seat, oriental coffee tables, a refrigerator, and a bed. My room was located at the end of a labyrinth of plants, statues, and camouflaged iron gates, under a pool house with ceilings so low I couldn't stand up without bumping my head. I added a stereo and black light, which distorted the room's dimensions; it became a haven for underage drinking and pot smoking. Some visitors bumped their heads on the ceiling while dancing. I walked with my lady guests to the big house to use the bathroom, and most men pissed on the plants away from my front door with the red glass. Some visitors fell into the fishpond on the way back through the maze to the street.

At work my strong math skills helped me learn two jobs in less time than most people took to learn one. Although my supervisor stayed on my case for being late, that didn't stop him from selecting me for advanced electrical and electronic training in preparation for future promotions. When I told coworkers I was going to quit my job to become a dental technician, many of them tried to convince me that I was making a career mistake. They brought in employment ads and showed me I would do better by keeping my job. But I had paid most of my tuition and signed a $1,000 student-loan promissory note for the balance. On my last day at work, they gave me a briefcase and an alarm clock.

Ron moved to Oakland the summer of 1969. He and Greg decided to share a three-bedroom furnished apartment in Berkeley with Greg's younger brother and two of his brother's best friends, both ex-Black Panthers, instead of getting their own apartment. After I showed up with two suitcases, albums, dishes, and a black light, everyone agreed I could sleep on the lumpy sofa for $50 a month. Greg's brother was the only one who didn't participate in political science class on Tuesdays. They called themselves the Collective and read Mao Tse-tung's *Four Essays on Philosophy*, Mao's Little Red Book, and other political writings. I attended when my schedule permitted.

I commuted from Berkeley to Career Academy School of Dental Technology located in the Fox Plaza Building on the corner of Ninth and Market in San Francisco. After class, I took the L streetcar to the Doggie Diner at Forty-seventh and Sloat, across the street from the San Francisco Zoo. I worked until midnight and arrived home after 2:00 am, only to return to school the same morning.

My employer relocated me to a Doggie Diner in El Cerrito, a small city near Berkeley, to help cut down on commute time. A much smaller diner, it barely had enough space between the grill and hot dog steam table for one person to work. One evening, the night manager, an overweight middle-aged white man, became overly friendly and crowded me near french fries bubbling in hot oil next to the grill. I pushed him back toward the hot dog steam table. The manager's left hand bounced off the steam table's hot cover, and his right hand grabbed for the cash register for balance. Customers looking through the glass laughed at the tussling cooks. He straightened his apron, looked back at me, and shouted, "I'll fix you!"

The next day he transferred me to a hostile Doggie Diner in Richmond located on the corner of Twenty-third and MacDonald. Foulmouthed white men gambled and drank liquor in the parking lot, just a couple of blocks from the Richmond police station. I commuted from Berkeley to San Francisco in the morning and to Richmond in the evening on AC Transit, the local public bus. After work, I would give the bus driver a large cup of coffee, and he paid my fifty-cent bus fare. I got off on San Pablo and University Avenue and walked approximately two miles uphill to my apartment on the corner of McGee and Addison near the Berkeley police station. I arrived home after 2:00 AM and got up that same morning after a few hours' sleep and commuted back to San Francisco. I carved wax teeth and studied dental concepts during my commute to work.

I turned down an opportunity to move into a studio apartment in the Fox Plaza Building. Instead I chose friendship and home-cooked meals, choices that were incongruent with attending Career Academy. Those long commutes coupled with little sleep compounded by attempts at partying caught up with me. I dropped out of school to pursue short-term bliss. By this time Ron had moved out, and I became his roommate in the penthouse, which was just up the street.

One evening two white men walked up to the Doggie Diner window.

"May I help you?" I asked. They didn't order anything.

"Aren't you from San Diego?" one of them asked. I became paranoid.

"Don't you go to dental school?" the other one asked. They knew too much about me. *Did they know I read Chairman Mao?* I called in sick the next day and never returned to work. Broke, I moved out of the penthouse apartment and onto a friend's floor. I became bitter and blamed my failures on the white lady from Saint Paul's Episcopal Church in San Diego. It was her fault for recommending Career Academy School of Dental Technology. I should have listened to my coworkers at North Island and kept my job.

*   *   *

My family moved from San Diego to the Philippines after I had moved to the Bay Area. Mother had asked me to meet her on their stopover at Travis Air Force Base just north of Oakland, en route to the Philippines. I didn't show up because I was too ashamed to tell her that I had dropped out of school and slept on a friend's floor. I was thankful for a place to sleep—rats tripping traps often woke me up. Many times I searched through grease-stained bags in the kitchen for burned barbecue doggie bone scraps to eat. I thought I was the only one until I met my roommate rummaging for meaty bones one morning.

After Mother arrived in the Philippines, she discovered Dad had a mistress. She returned to her parents' once-segregated oasis, Chesapeake Gardens, with four children and no financial support. She went back to school, earned a certificate in culinary science, and became a cook for Norfolk Public Schools. She then forever referred to her husband, James, as PH1, photographer first class, a name my brothers and sisters would use instead of Daddy.

CHAPTER 5

Decision Time

MY NERVES TREMBLED as my large frame lay poised on a slim gurney before entering the extremely small test cylinder of the multiton MRI machine. I wasn't ready for the loud banging sound every ten seconds as the machine inched me inside. Fortunately, my tumor was in my tongue, which shortened each test since only my head and shoulders had to enter the machine's magnetic flux field. I was spared the agony of long-term tight confinement, although the deafening noise rattled me.

Dr. Watson's staff had arranged my consultation with Dr. Bruce Rice, a tall slender man who typically wore a white short-sleeve shirt with a tie and gray slacks. His office was near the University of California at Berkeley, a few blocks west of Telegraph Avenue near People's Park, an old visible link to Berkeley's Free Speech Movement of the 1960s.

I completed the usual first-visit forms upon arrival and sat speechless next to Monica while she gazed at magazines.

"Mr. and Mrs. Green, please follow me," said the nurse.

I stood first, extended my hand to help Monica. We proceeded to a small examination room distinguished by a black-leather-and-chrome chair in the center and large pictures of nasal passages and ear cavities on the wall. I saw Monica's attention drawn to the exposed lightbulb without the typical protective shadelike lens next to the chair as she entered the room and sat under the nasal passage picture. I sat in the chair, and from her vantage point, I must have looked like a political prisoner awaiting interrogation.

A no-nonsense-looking man entered the quaint room and sat next to me on a short swivel stool, with his back to Monica.

"Hello, my name is Gerald Green, and behind you is my wife Monica Green," I said. I saw Monica's eyes beaming.

"Hello, Dr. Rice," Monica said in a don't-ignore-me tone. He turned toward her.

"Good afternoon, Mrs. Green," he said. The tiny examination room seemed to be designed for two-way conversations and made the threesome awkward. Monica resigned herself to reading her book until she noticed his degrees on the wall.

"I see you went to medical school at the University of Nebraska," she said.

He turned his attention to her and smiled.

"Yes," he said. Monica relaxed her facial muscles.

"My sister's son is on their football team," she said.

Dr. Rice stopped reviewing my reports and looked up at her.

"Didn't they win top national ranking?" he asked.

"Yes," she replied. "My sister completed law school at Creighton in Omaha, Nebraska." He acknowledged her with a slight nod and returned his attention to me. It seemed to me that he was more comfortable now that Monica had broken the ice between us.

"When did you first notice your lesion?" he asked.

"My dentist, Dr. Perry, discovered it during a routine visit approximately two months ago," I said.

He firmly placed both hands on the base of my neck and pressed.

"What was his recommendation?" he asked.

"Dr. Perry referred me to another dentist, Dr. Murphy."

He wrote in my file. "Who did your biopsy?" he asked.

"Dr. Murphy," I said.

Dr. Rice erupted. "A dentist did this to you! They aren't surgeons." Monica looked up from her book.

"A surgeon wouldn't have cut up your tongue like this," he said. I sat quietly, looking into Monica's eyes for relief. He lowered a metal shield with a hole in the center over his eye.

"I need you to open your mouth as wide as possible. This may be a little uncomfortable," he said. He pulled the lightbulb closer to the side of my face and pressed his latex-covered right index finger into the right side of my mouth just below my tongue, deep into the floor, until I flinched. Then the same prodding finger pushed deep into the left side of the floor of my mouth.

"Mr. Green, please stick out your tongue." I complied with his request. Dr. Rice pushed his index finger onto my tongue while holding it with gauze.

"Does that hurt?" he asked. His finger moved toward the lesion area. I jumped a little and retracted my tongue from his grip.

"Yes!"

"It's difficult to distinguish between the lesion and scar tissue from the biopsy," he said, uttering just above a whisper. His looks of concern seemed to acknowledge my pain.

"I don't understand why people go to dentists for surgery," he said. I sensed some sort of professional turf rivalry. Dr. Rice grabbed a small-diameter mirror extended on a thin three-inch stainless steel rod from a tray of assorted medical instruments and held it near the naked lightbulb as if he were heating it. I looked at him oddly.

"Open your mouth wide, please. This will not hurt." I opened my mouth as wide as I could. Dr. Rice took a wooden tongue depressor and pressed on my tongue. He moved the heated mirror toward the rear of my mouth and said, "Say the letter A."

I awkwardly said, "Aaaaaaaa . . ."

He removed the mirror and said, "Thanks, Mr. Green." He then felt my upper neck area. His long, firm fingers gripped below my jaw and felt odd as they brushed aside my beard. He later told me he was checking my lymph node glands. He uttered, "Ummm," with head nodding slightly up and down; and his fingers paused as if they could discriminate between good from bad tissues. He pushed his swivel stool around, looked at us.

"Mr. and Mrs. Green, my examination confirms your tumor is a good candidate for radiation therapy," Dr. Rice said. It felt like we just stepped on another bread crumb toward recovery.

"Is that good news?" I asked.

"Yes, radiation therapy tends to be less intrusive than surgery," he said. I saw hope in Monica's face.

"What's the next step?" I asked. He looked at my chart and wrote some notes. "I'll refer you to Dr. Myles Lampenfeld, a radiation oncologist."

"What about side effects?" I asked.

"You should ask Dr. Lampenfeld," he said. He closed my chart, gave us polite eye contact.

"Mr. Green, is there anything else I can do for you?" he asked. I had almost forgotten about my earaches, which sometimes exceeded the pain in my tongue.

"I've been experiencing periodic acute pain in my left ear," I said. He moved toward me, leaned forward, and looked deep into each ear with a small black conelike device.

"You have a very nasty infection," he said. He reached for a stainless steel tube approximately two and one-half inches long. It was connected to a thin black rubber hose, leading to a small jar from a pump. He gently placed the tube into my ear and turned on the pump, which sucked a small amount of liquid wax substance from my left ear and then my right ear.

"You have bacteria and excessive fluid. That's caused your pain," said Dr. Rice. Monica took deep breaths as she looked at the brown fluid trickle into the bottle next to the pump.

"You have fluid in the right ear too. You must keep them dry." I heard what he said, but my mind was fixed on using our swimming pool, which we had just repaired. The pool was the key reason I wanted to buy the house.

"Is there a way I can go swimming?" I asked. He looked at me in disbelief.

"Didn't you hear me?"

"Yes, I heard you, but I've been waiting since May for completion of major pool repairs," I said.

"You're not serious!"

"Yes, I am. What about earplugs?"

"Those things don't keep water out of your ears," he said, looking at me. "The best way is to rub some Vaseline into a small piece of cotton and place that into your ears. You should do that when taking a shower."

"So I can swim."

"No, I don't recommend any swimming." He stood and shook his head. "I want to see you in a week. Please make a follow-up appointment at the front desk."

*   *   *

I forgot about the three-hour time difference when I called my brother.

"Hello, David. How are you and Willa?"

"Who is this? Is this Jerry?" I felt his outrage.

"Yes, brother, it's me. I apologize for the early-morning call, but it has been a while since we talked." I was trying to build up the nerve to discuss my diagnosis when he said, "You know, Jerry . . . Mother has been undergoing some gall bladder tests." Listening to him talk about Mother's illness help me gain strength.

"What's her status?" I asked.

"There are a couple more tests they want to do, but they had to postpone them until her blood pressure stabilized," he said. He sounded more awake.

"OK . . . Any idea when?" I asked.

"It'll be at least another month," he said. Our conversation had warmed up my courage.

"David, I've had a few medical examinations too . . . I was diagnosed with tongue cancer."

"What did you say?"

"I was diagnosed with tongue cancer. Fortunately, it was detected early." I heard David's heavy breath of relief. "One of my doctors recommends radiation therapy. I'll meet with a radiation oncologist next Tuesday." The line went silent.

"How are you holding up?" David asked.

"It has been a rough couple of weeks."

"I can't imagine," he said. I felt the same about him. I couldn't imagine all the pressure on his shoulders, dealing with Mother.

"I've been traveling an emotional roller-coaster ride," I said.

"When does your treatment start?" he asked.

"I'll find out next week. You know, David . . . the last thing Mother needs to hear is I have cancer." My phone hand had grown numb.

"You got a point. That'll just give her something else to worry about and keep up her blood pressure," he said. I switched hands.

"You're right. We shouldn't burden her with this now," I said.

CHAPTER 6

Baby Teeth

CHARLES GAINED A few ounces; and his physician, Dr. Bean, requested a follow-up.

Monica took Charles to child care, and I went to my doctors' appointment. I explained to them that other than periodic pains and a slight loss of appetite, I felt good. I appreciated their attention, but back-to-back appointments dampened my enthusiasm about my MBA interview. Although Dr. Watson thought considering the MBA program was too optimistic, I believed it was important I follow through with the interview and decide later if I would attend or not. An MBA would help me find a bridge from corporate middle manager to entrepreneur, if I lost my job because PG&E was downsizing to stay competitive in a deregulated environment.

Unfortunately, after two promotions and numerous performance awards, my job responsibilities stopped increasing, which convinced me my interview was crucial to survive in a lean middle management position in corporate America. I chose the executive MBA program because it was set up for business practitioners with emphasis on experience, but I knew my poor undergraduate grades would draw attention.

My mind raced back in time as I drove to the MBA interview. I thought about my sixth-grade teacher, Bob Matthews, an African American ex-army man who served as my surrogate father when Dad was away. Mr. Matthews believed in me and helped me achieve excellence. Mr. Matthews became the first black male that I wanted to emulate outside my extended family. Like many sixth graders, my knowledge of careers was very narrow. I was not sure what I wanted to be; I thought an engineer was the person that operated a train. It is rather ironic that I became a mechanical engineer two decades later; and for the past thirteen years, I had worked with black youth helping them become more aware of their rich heritage of black engineers, inventors, and scientists. I did this as a down payment on my personal debt to Mr. Matthews for helping me release my greatness hidden under layers of self-doubt.

"Good afternoon. Please have a seat," said the receptionist. "They are running a little behind." I sat and thought about different ways to respond to questions, knowing this would be an uphill struggle. Thirteen years ago, PG&E employment representatives returned my employment request with "you lack qualifications and experiences." I knew they were referring to my grades. Fortunately, I received an invitation for an interview from PG&E after they received a letter from the Concentrated Employment Project of the California Department of Rehabilitation. I had a bad knee, and the state had provided me resources throughout college and written letters in my behalf after I graduated.

All I wanted was a chance to compete. But I left three interviewers with what seemed like doubting faces. I hoped they saw what Mr. Matthews discovered, my ability to achieve excellence.

Just three weeks prior, Monica and I traveled this same peaceful circuitous route home from Saint Mary's College with illusions of tranquility. I had none this time, and without Monica's fear of heights to slow me down, the five-cylinder turbo diesel belched black smoke as I sped along the twisting roads. Quietly, an invisible society kept calling me when I accelerated through curves. One of my best friends, Ron, who played college football and was the picture of good health, was inducted into this invisible society, a silent order of survivors, when a cancerous tumor the size of a golf ball was detected in his thigh. We had met in 1967 when our families comprised the few African Americans living in military housing camouflaged as indigenous homes in the Pacific Beach area of San Diego, California. Some of our neighbors didn't appreciate our presence and called us niggers and flipped us the finger.

Shortly after I was diagnosed with cancer, Monica, Charles, and I visited Ron and his wife, Jeanie, in blistering hot Winters, California, just outside of Sacramento. While Monica and Jeanie entertained Charles under a cool oak tree, Ron and I swam and reminisced about the past. We recalled the night in December 1969 in our Berkeley penthouse apartment when we celebrated the announcements of our very high Vietnam draft lottery numbers.

No one then ever thought either of us would contract cancer. Ron was given a fifty-fifty chance of surviving cancer one year, and I felt good helping him celebrate life ten years later. Talking to him gave me hope that

I too would survive, and with that fresh hope, I met with my radiation oncologists.

The invisible world became opaque as I sat waiting for Dr. Lampenfeld with other patients, some bald. Unlike waiting to see Drs. Watson and Rice, I felt kinship with this group because we all shared a common diagnosis—cancer. With proud faces, not cheerful or sad, they walked in and sat before entering a door to radiation treatment, one that I too would enter in five weeks.

"Mr. Green, please follow me," said the nurse. I stood and followed her through the door to an examination room where she took my blood pressure and weight.

"Dr. Lampenfeld will be with you momentarily," she said. I searched the empty white walls before Dr. Myles Lampenfeld entered the room.

"Dr. Rice called me and requested I examine you for possible radiation therapy," he said. I discovered one year later while reviewing Social Security records during my appeal for benefits that Dr. Rice had described me to Dr. Lampenfeld as a forty-six-year-old black executive with a lesion on the mid third of the tongue with moderately differentiated squamous cell carcinoma. He'd promoted me from an engineer to an executive, something that had eluded me to date, and maybe that helped facilitated my excellent treatment. Dr. Lampenfeld sat next to me and proceeded to ask the usual list of questions. I kept Tinman's activities from my answers. He felt my neck before asking me to open wide. His examination was short compared to Dr. Rice's.

"Good news," he said. "Your tumor seems to be less than four centimeters and is classified as a T2N0." I frowned in confusion.

"What's that?" I asked. He explained that the T was for tumor and numeric value usually varied from zero to four depending on its size. A T0 meant no evidence of primary tumor while a T1 and T2 are small tumors, and a T3 is greater than four centimeters. A T4 is a tumor that has invaded adjacent structures like bone and muscle. The N is for lymph node, and the 0 means no regional lymph node metastasis.

"What does all of this mean?" I asked.

"Since there is no metastasis, implant therapy is a good companion treatment with the external radiation beam," he said. He saw the confusion on my face.

"Implant therapy, or brachytherapy, consists of inserting small plastic catheters around the tumor, then running a radiation source through them." He went on to explain that the procedure took a week and that it was considered standard procedure.

"Will you do it?" I asked.

"No, Dr. Jeffrey Demanes will perform your procedure," he said. "Normally we recommend external radiation first, but because of the location of your tumor we recommend that you receive brachytherapy first."

I looked blankly into space, and Dr. Lampenfeld saw my shoulders slump. He spoke loudly.

"And the good news is we think the combined treatment has an 80 percent chance of killing all of the cancer cells." My head snapped up. I remembered Ron's 50 percent chance and felt great about my prognosis.

"You will suffer a lost of taste. However, most clients regain about 90 percent," he said. He wrote in my chart. "Your salivary glands are in the radiation field, and they may temporarily fail to provide adequate secretion. You will experience possible dry mouth. That condition may be permanent." I looked at him.

"What does that mean?" I asked.

"Your mouth will remain permanently dry, requiring constant lubrication."

I sensed his uneasiness telling me some of my body parts would not function anymore, but our eyes somehow locked in friendly exchanges during our discussion—besides, life is better than a few failed body parts. He continued, "Some of the other acute side effects are dermatitis, which is an inflammation of the skin. You will experience mucositis, an inflammation of the inside of your mouth, some localized hair loss, and general body fatigue."

"You sure know how to rain on a parade. You mean I'll lose my beard."

"Yes," he said and continued writing without looking up.

"I've had a beard for over twenty years. Most people including my wife don't even know what my face looks like." He continued writing and nodded his head.

"Yes, most of the hair on the right side of your face will fall out as we proceed with the treatment," he said.

"I'll have hair only on the left side . . ."

"You may, but some of that will fall out too." I hid fear behind my beard, and now I had to part with my shield.

"Any other side effects?" I asked.

"You may suffer from long-term tooth decay. You should see your dentist for an evaluation and fluoride treatment." I was mentally exhausted from hearing consequences and things to do.

"I have an appointment with my dentist, Dr. Perry, today," I said. He looked surprised.

"Dr. Curtis Perry, I know him," he said. His tall slender frame stood. "Our sons are in the same baseball league." Although he treated me with respect, just hearing that he knew my dentist gave me a much-needed emotional lift as I left his subterranean office in the Alta Bates Comprehensive Cancer Center. Dr. Lampenfeld had become the third physician to join my dream team of three medical doctors and two dentists.

*   *   *

At my last dental visit, Dr. Perry retrofitted my partials so they wouldn't slip, but increasing pain prevented me from wearing them. I thanked him as I always did for detecting my lesion early. However, I sensed he felt guilty somehow about his discovery. *How strange*, I thought, as I sat waiting for the receptionist. She came in and directed me to a room with the familiar low, elongated banana-shaped examining chair. I bent my knees, climbed in, and attempted pleasant thoughts; but my mind kept returning to radiation side effects as I waited for Dr. Perry. Time stalled. My mounting apprehension was interrupted.

"Hello, Gerald. How are you?" Dr. Perry asked.

"Not so good. Dr. Lampenfeld just explained some of the possible side effects of radiation."

Nervous energy vibrated in my left hand as I pulled at some of the long chin portion of my beard. My right hand held the arm of the chair tightly, and my eyes meandered, avoiding Dr. Perry.

"Myles Lampenfeld, it's a small world. Our sons play ball in the same league," he said. My hand released the arm of the chair, and I looked at him for the first time. He smiled. I attempted one, but my lips were locked together. He asked me to open wide. I licked my lips and took a deep swallow before complying.

"Gerald! You have three baby teeth," he said with a chuckle. "They'll never survive your radiation treatment." That wasn't funny to me, but I could appreciate his humor—a forty-six-year-old man with three baby teeth—God had already blessed me with dark brown skin, a flattened nose, gapped front teeth, knock-knee, and now cancer. My emotions rose and ebbed as he explained in detail how my mouth might never heal if my baby teeth weren't pulled before the radiation treatment.

"How many teeth will I have left after you pull those?" I asked. He looked on his computer screen next to my chair and counted.

"Twelve."

"Ain't that something? A whole dozen, I think Charles has three," I said.

"Who is Charles?" he asked.

"Our son," I said with lifted sprits. He stopped typing on the keyboard.

"I didn't know you and Monica had a son. Congratulations! How old is he?"

"He turned one year old last month."

"That sounds great," he said. "Now I need you to keep your mouth open. I'm going to give you a little topical sedative."

"It won't hurt, will it?" I asked.

CHAPTER 7

The Yes Game

THE COMMUTER TRAFFIC constantly stalled. I shifted gears every mile or so as I drove my red radioless 1978 Ford F-100 truck to pick up Charles. His smile greeted me as I entered the day care facility and helped release my built-up tension and anxiety.

"Hi, Charles, how are you doing?" His smile grew larger as he kicked his feet and crawled toward me. He babbled without a care. I wished my life was as innocent.

While driving home he began grunting. I saw him squeeze his lips together and close his eyes as his little body contorted. "Charles, you're making *stink stink in the wink wink*." Normally, Monica and I didn't talk baby talk to him, but like many parents, I sometimes lapsed. Saying phrases like "stink stink in the wink wink" made cleaning up his mess less of a chore.

At home I changed him and asked, "Charles, are you hungry?" His head turned toward me as he tried to mouth an answer. His verbal response wasn't clear, but his body language said, "Yes, feed me, Daddy."

I turned on Maze's *Back to Basics* and bounced Charles on my lap while warming up his dinner of rice with sautéed prawns and broccoli. The smooth sounds of Maze and Frankie Beverly helped lower my apprehension about cancer's unknown journey and helped me focus on feeding Charles. Food drooled from his fat golden brown cheeks until he refused to swallow any more.

"Charles, did you enjoy your dinner?"

"Da . . . da, moo . . . ," he seemed to have said.

"I hope so," I said. He smiled again without answering as I wiped his face and hand clean. We retired to the family room, where we played the yes game. I wanted Charles to hear the word *yes* associated with love, books, and other positive objects. I would say, "Yes, Charles, Mommy and Daddy love you. Yes, Charles, Daddy will read you a book. Yes, Charles, you may read the book to Daddy. Yes, Charles, you may go to the library. And yes, Charles, you may do more homework."

Charles's brown eyes darted around. Maze continued to play in the background. I hoped these yes deposits into his emotional bank account, paid dividends before any withdrawals like "No, Charles, stop doing that." Making his deposits reminded me that I must keep a healthy emotional outlook, so I played the yes game.

Yes, my radiation treatment will succeed. Yes, we will survive this together.

"Thank you, Charles," I said. "Daddy needed 'yes' deposits too."

Monica entered the kitchen from the garage. Her smile radiated and helped ease the fading effects of my local anesthesia.

"Hi, baby. Rough day?" I asked.

"I'm OK. The day wasn't bad, you know, just the same old office politics," she said. "I'm tired of my boss telling the same old stale male jokes. Gee, you and Charles look relaxed. I want a hug." I stood up with Charles, and we all hugged.

"We were playing the yes game," I said. Monica chimed in, "Yes, I love you, Gerald and Charles," before leaving to change clothes. Charles and I gathered a few books and settled in the living room. I turned off the music before sitting down to read, not knowing that a year later, my radiation therapy would temporarily rob me of that simple pleasure. We heard Monica in the kitchen. I read *Golden Bear*. It became our favorite bedtime book because it ended with the little boy tucked in bed. Monica joined us after eating, and she read the poems from *Nathaniel Talking* until Charles fell asleep. We tucked him in his crib and returned to the living room, where we sat on the floor close to each other with our backs against the sofa.

"So how was your day?" Monica asked.

"It was mixed. I met with Dr. Lampenfeld this morning. He was younger than I'd anticipated," I said. Her face returned a supporting gesture beyond a smile.

"Oh, what did he say?" she asked. We sat for what seemed like hours discussing my options.

"Baby, can you come with me this Thursday for my 2:00 pm appointment with Dr. Demanes at?" I asked.

"Ah, I have to meet with some people flying in from South Carolina." I hadn't expected her answer, but I was ready to move forward. I had her spirit coupled with my optimism. We embraced, and I felt better.

We moved our conversation to the patio and sat in the deep green wrought iron swinging love seat, facing the pool. Monica and I swung, looking at the tall pine trees behind the pool with the setting sun flickering through their branches. I dozed off and recalled when I was a little boy swinging in the hot summer heat on my great-granddaddy's porch with my cousins. We sipped lemonade and counted the few cars that passed on the dirt road in front of the house for entertainment, because my great aunt didn't allow us to listen to the radio on Sundays.

"Gerald, wake up," Monica said. "Have you given any thought to my cousin's twenty-fifth wedding anniversary?"

"What did you say?" I asked.

"Barbara and Nelson's wedding anniversary. They're going to renew their wedding vows, then celebrate," she said.

"OK, but I don't think I'll be up for the celebration."

"Why?" she asked.

"I don't feel like partying. I'm not sure about this implant therapy."

"But didn't Dr. Lampenfeld say an 80 percent chance of success?" Monica said.

"Yeah, but I want to hear what Dr. Demanes has to say."

"Aw, don't worry," she said. "Perhaps we should go back inside, just in case Charles wakes up." And the sun hid behind the clouds.

"Monica, I need your help to cover the pool."

We unrolled the blue plastic cover on the aluminum spool located in the shallow end of the pool. She turned the wheel, and I pulled it toward the deep end of the pool, trapping the escaping misty heat. I took one last look before following her into the house.

"I checked on the baptism schedule last Sunday for Charles. They have slots available, in August and November," Monica said. I wasn't paying attention; I could almost feel the warm water lapping against me as if I were swimming.

"What did you say, baby?"

"Should we pick August or November?" Monica said.

"Well, August is definitely out. How soon must you confirm a date?" I asked.

"I don't know. I'll check Sunday. Do you want to come?"

"I'm not sure," I said. Knowing all the time that I didn't want to go, I felt uncomfortable at Saint Paschal Baylon Catholic Church's mostly white congregation. It brought back bad memories of blatant racism in the

Episcopal church in Lexington Park, Maryland, and my hypocritical behavior in San Diego, where as a teenager I attended church with hangovers from partying the night before.

Monica selected Saint Paschal Baylon because of its location and school. However, it was the wholesomeness of the pastor and congregation that persuaded her to join. I supported her decision, and we attended some services together, but I wasn't ready to convert to Catholicism, and I couldn't let my past interfere with Charles's baptism plans. We needed God's help.

*   *   *

Money became a strong incentive to return to work. It had been nineteen days since my cancer diagnosis, yet I'd taken nine days off because of periodic acute pain and doctors' appointments. I had approximately sixty-three days of combined sick leave and vacation days remaining, enough to last through the middle of December. If I remained unable to work at that point, my income would drop to only $336 a week until I qualified for long-term disability, which would pay half of my gross pay.

Managing PG&E projects grew burdensome. Thoughts about my implant-therapy treatment ranged from *What is it?* to *How does it work?* Apprehension about my appointment coupled with recurring pain rendered me useless. I went home at noon to visit my new companion—sleep. My afternoon nap stole the evening. I didn't remember Monica and Charles coming home. I woke up slightly when her warm body rubbed next to mine, when she whispered, "Good night."

The next day I woke up with Charles. Monica and I were evolving into tag team parents. I dressed and fed him while she slept. She woke up as I finished packing his bag, and we hugged her before leaving.

"I know you must still be tired from last night," she said.

"Thanks for not waking me up," I said. Charles turned his little head back and forth, throwing toothy smiles at us.

"Say 'Good morning, Mommy,'" I said to him. He looked at me and Monica.

"Are you guys ready to go?" she asked and took him into her arms.

"Yeah, baby, he's all packed. Wish me luck at Dr. Demanes." Monica said good-bye, winked, and blew kisses, and drove Charles to the sitter.

I arrived a half hour late for work and worked a half a day before traveling back to Oakland in the midday heat. I parked near Merritt Hospital emergency entrance, close to Dr. Demanes's cramped space, which was less ornate than Dr. Lampenfeld's subterranean waiting area made with marble columns stretching to ground-level skylights, peering at manicured gardens. Ironically, near both entrances, clearly marked CANCER TREATMENT, groups of cigarette smokers congregated. *Are they blind, or are we cancer patients invisible?*

Stealthily, I waded through their smoke and indifference to meet Dr. Demanes. His examination started with the standard questions, and he thoroughly checked my mouth and neck. Unlike the others, he completed his examination by inserting a fiber optic scope through my nose.

"Uh-huh, that looks good . . . now, hold still, Mr. Green," Dr. Demanes said. He maneuvered the thin flexible snakelike device up around my nasal passage and down my throat, rendering me speechless. "Now hold still, you're doing great. Here it comes. There, I got it." He pulled the long black segmented device from my nose and throat. He sensed my uneasiness and immediately reassured me that a combination of implant therapy and external treatment was the best course of action.

"What exactly is implant therapy?" I asked.

"It's a procedure where I'll insert approximately twenty to thirty thin hollow polyethylene catheters through your tongue and neck while you are under general anesthesia." I looked at him in disbelief.

"I must immobilize your tongue by sewing it to the floor of your mouth, and if excessive swelling occurs, we'll perform a tracheotomy," Dr. Demanes said. My heart seemed to flutter with each word.

"You'll probably need between six to eight treatments and require a minimum of five days in the hospital," he said. My breath quickened; *Just five days,* I thought. I wanted reassurance and took some comfort in examining his numerous degrees and certificates around his office.

"You said something about twenty to thirty catheters," I stammered.

"Yes, they are connected to a device called an afterloader," he said.

"A what?" I asked.

"It's a machine we programmed with your tumor profile, and each treatment consists of it delivering a predetermined amount of a radioactive iridium-192 source to selected locations around your tumor." I winced. It didn't sound appealing, but it was better than the alternative. I recalled Dr. Murphy's solution of cutting off half my tongue and thought Dr. Demanes's approach was less dramatic and disfiguring.

"I understand your apprehension," he said. "You are fortunate we got to your tumor early." I forced a half smile.

"My partner, Dr. Rodriguez, underwent implant therapy for a tumor in his back, and he has fully recovered," he said. My smile grew.

"We have had great success treating T2N0 tumors at the base of the tongue." My heart rate seemed to return to normal, and my breathing slowed. I was starting to feel good about my choice and chances for survival.

"There's an 80 to 85 percent chance of total tumor elimination," Dr. Demanes said. I tugged at my beard.

"That sounds great. But a lot of this depends on your three-dimensional computer model and its ability to mimic real time," I said. He looked surprised.

"What platform are you using, and what safeguards does your program have to protect me from a radiation overdose?" I asked. He stopped writing and took a long look across the desk at me.

"We perform only implant therapy here and have been doing so for fifteen years," he said in an affirming voice.

"Fifteen years?" I echoed to myself in relief.

"Yes, and we use a Silicon Graphics workstation and a Nucletron remote afterloading system, the best equipment. Plus our staff is fully trained in all operational phases and safety protocol procedures," he said.

"OK," I said. I had a big ear-to-ear smile and thought, *Ah . . . yes, Silicon Graphics' hardware*. They make the best computers for simulating real time.

"What's a remote afterloading system?" I asked.

"It's the key to your treatment and our safety. We retreat behind a lead shield, and the afterloader runs very thin radioactive needles through the catheter implants around your tumor," he said.

Something about the inflection of his voice and willingness to discuss details about equipment and procedures, along with his numerous wall-mounted degrees and certifications, convinced me that he could deliver the first phase of my treatment strategy. Dr. Lampenfeld's external treatment would complete the tandem tag team radiation attack on my tumor. Dr. Rice would later give me a third-party evaluation of their workmanship while Dr. Watson orchestrated approval for all procedures.

I relied heavily upon Dr. Watson's insight and guidance throughout my treatment, and I would grow to trust them all.

CHAPTER 8

Implant Treatment

I HAD DRIVEN to Summit Medical Center many times to visit Dr. Demanes when the sidewalks were full of people hurrying for sandwiches, chips, and drinks, but never before predawn birdsongs. This morning, Monica and I drove by empty liquor stores with blinking colored neon signs in vacant twilight spaces, traffic signals controlling empty streets. The light turned red. Monica sat quietly, held my hand waiting, while trash swirled and danced in the wind. The light turned green, and Monica gently rubbed my forearm, as I pulled into the parking garage.

We walked together holding hands like newlyweds leaving the chapel and approached the elevator's entrance to the hospital. Neither one of us said much, just locked hands as we walked toward presurgery reception. I opened the door and was surprised to see a room full of people, some with expressions of dismay and concern, and others like me—just plain old scared. After I completed the paperwork, I sat next to Monica.

"Mr. and Mrs. Green, please follow me," a nurse called out. We stood and followed her through a door into a very large room with thin white sheets sectioning off areas where people were lying down. Some were alone, others with a friend or loved one sitting next to them.

"Here, Mrs. Green, you may sit there. Mr. Green, please follow me," a nurse said. Monica sat in a chair behind the sheets.

"You can change in there," she said. She gave me a couple large plastic bags for my clothes and valuables. I changed into my hospital gown, then returned and stretched out on the bed next to Monica.

A different nurse explained how she was going to insert a needle in the top of my hand for an IV. She had aged pinkish freckled hands, soft and warm. She slowly stroked the back of my hand before inserting the IV. I tightly closed my lips and eyes anticipating the needle's pain.

"Relax now, relax," she said, before penetrating my skin. My hand throbbed and burned. She pushed deeper; and my inflamed nerves vacated tranquility, pushing me into mental space away from patients waiting for scalpels, needles, and clamps. I opened my eyes and looked away, beyond the white translucent curtains separating me from others before 6:00 am surgery. She looked down and gave me a grandma smile.

"Now, that didn't hurt, did it?" she asked. Her tender hands started to absorb the burning heat radiating from my aching hand, before releasing me pain free, with a fresh IV plug in place, ready to receive life-sustaining fluids.

"Yeah, a little," I said with a sigh. The anesthesiologist entered.

"Have you had anything to drink or eat in the last twelve hours?" he asked.

"No."

The anesthesiologist explained the potential drug side effects and then requested me to count backward from a hundred: one hundred, ninety-nine, ninety-eight, and ninety-seven. I thought about Dr. Demanes's warning, *I must insert a plastic breathing tube in your trachea if swelling occurs.* My body grew warm. I saw Monica's face fade into darkness.

*　　*　　*

An orderly pushed a quivering body on the gurney, with needlelike porcupine quills extending from his right cheek. It was me—Gerald. People turned their heads, stared, and probably thought, "What the shit?" The brother pushing the gurney only shrugged his shoulders and kept on. He slowly moved Gerald into a large empty hospital-white room toward a life-support station adjacent to a wall with an assortment of colored lines.

The body on the gurney began to thaw from his drug-induced sleep, alone with splitting nerves that forced his lower extremities to twitch. First, his right leg jerked about like wounded prey shot from the sky and, after hitting the ground, attempting to fly away. His left hand grabbed at empty air before it fell. His wounded body had started to detoxify, like junkies at night without another fix. His dreamworld was interrupted by a mucus-clogged throat, which squeezed air from his trachea that rattled in his chest. Each breath's ebb was followed by violent kicks that rocked his gurney and jeopardized the connections to the machines that sustained his life.

Gerald's tongue had been sewn to the floor of his mouth to prevent movement of a rainbow of thirty thin catheters lacing tissue around the tumor buried deep in his tongue. His eyes flickered behind tightly closed eyelids. Cramping waves washed misery over his face and down his legs. Pain shuddered everywhere. Helplessly, he dove into mental pools of tranquility to shed his torment, and his soul swam away in search of rest.

He opened his eyes that evening alone in a room with a white ceiling. A nurse walked toward him. She saw his probing eyes before stretching over him to silence the alarm. His torso gyrated, screaming for help.

"I can see you have been through a lot. I know you can't talk, but I hope you can understand me," she said. She looked into his eyes for some form of acknowledgment. He flickered and blinked his eyes, not understanding why his body hurt. Her hand took his and held it, checking his pulse.

"Now I'm gonna take good care of you," she said. She went about tucking him under the covers he had kicked off. "You need something to relax those muscles, before you tear up your gurney. I'll be right back."

Alone again, he slipped into the sea with angels. They protected his mind as the anesthesiologist's drug effect lapsed and schools of sharks sank their teeth into him. He couldn't defend himself, and tears rolled through a field of catheters onto his sheet. The axis of misery shifted from his lower body to his head. It seemed to expand with each tick of the plain-numbered clock on the white windowless wall. The ticktocks echoed off his helium balloonlike face with plastic tubes pricking his right side. Unfortunately, those pinholes didn't deflate his agony, and his eyes retreated deeper into their sockets in search for relief. He could only look up slightly to his left and couldn't see the nurse as she entered the room.

"I'm back," she said. His heart throbbed hearing her voice. "I got something to calm your body." She gently rolled him onto his side, and he grunted in an attempt to help.

"That's right, just a little more . . . there, got it." She moved around to his backside, lifted his gown, grabbed an alcohol wipe, and cleaned a patch of flesh. She squeezed his buttocks and stuck him with a needle.

"How was that? That didn't hurt, did it?" she asked. "You'll start feeling better soon." She walked around into his view, smiling.

"I'll be right back. You rest now, the medicine will relax you," she said. She walked out of the room, leaving him motionless for the first time since he arrived. He rested in his new quiet space, slipping back to a dimension void of spasms, time, and feelings. He awoke and thought he heard voices.

"Where should I take him?" someone asked.

"Oh, he goes to room 300 in intensive care. I'll be right there to help you transfer his equipment," the nurse said. She cast doubtful eyes, as if wondering, *Where do they find these guys?*

"Wait, don't touch that. Let me do that," she said. He stepped back from the gurney and waited for instructions, for a task he had done alone hundreds of times.

"OK, now first take the oxygen bottle and place under the gurney. I'll disconnect the line from the wall and connect it to the bottle. Do you understand?"

"Yes," he said. He bent down and placed the bottle in its rack. He had done this without assistance earlier but didn't make a fuss and followed her instructions. They continued their lopsided teamwork.

"He's yours, take him to room 300."

He pushed Gerald into the hall and accelerated toward the elevator, which made the catheters and feeding tube down Gerald's nose tingle. Gerald didn't know if they were going up or down, but they exited on what seemed like a cobblestoned road. *Somebody please tell him to slow down,* Gerald thought, but he sped up, blind to Gerald's suffering. Gerald replaced those bouncing vibrating pricks with pleasant thoughts about his grandparents' church, where he had learned his ABCs and manners when he was a little boy. Granddaddy died when Gerald was sixteen, and he and his cousins remembered how they each almost dropped him as they carried the casket holding his body from Shiloh Baptist Church to the long black limousine. They drove him sixty-five miles, followed by a parade of cars, to Chapel on the Hill Baptist Church in Norlina, North Carolina, in 1964. They did the same for Grandmother ten years later.

Gerald didn't understand then how his grandparents had protected him from the ills of a separate and an unequal society. Those emotional scars festered over time and transformed into anger. Because in the mid-'70s Chevron promoted Gerald to a retail sales representative who was responsible for collecting money from Chevron gas stations in four Bay Area counties, until they then forced him to take his vacation after he had trained his white vacation replacement. While he was on vacation, they demoted him back to pumping gas and gave the white man his retail sales representative job.

Gerald arrived safely to intensive care, but mentally his past haunted him.

*   *   *

"Help, I can't breathe," I wanted to say. "I can't clear my . . ." I couldn't move my tongue, and I choked on an extra thick blob of mucus, which made my chest muscles tighten with each attempt to breathe, making me faint with every effort.

Help, I can't breathe! I thought silently. No one responded to my fading, muted cries, so I flapped my arms and slapped my bed to gain the attention from people moving just outside my door. I saw them, but they ignored me as they moved about, checking paperwork. I wanted to say, "Look at me! I can't breathe! I can't breathe! Help! Someone please help me," but couldn't speak. I remembered saying this over and over again to myself, as I slipped back into my dreamy place filled with fond childhood memories. I awoke to see two pairs of eyes scanning my voiceless shell.

"Remove his tube," a short thin woman said to the olive-toned woman. The nurse of color approached me saying, "This may hurt a little." She slowly began pulling the L-shaped trachea connector out of my throat. It made a sound like a cork popping out of a bottle once she had it out. The pressure that was once trapped burst out and vigorously vibrated my fingernails. I clenched the side of the bed for relief and gasped for air, staring into the blue eyes of the thin nurse. She then sprayed a saline-tasting solution into my trachea.

"Cough," she said. Before I could, she stepped behind me, and the nurse of color stood off to my side. I took a deep congested, rattling breath. I felt a salty tingling sensation before huffing and pushing all the air from my lungs, along with flying blobs of spattering mucus, until I swallowed unobstructed air. I breathed in fresh hospital air in my white-walled room filled with ticking, echoing sterile machines.

"He has strong lungs," the nurse of color said before pressing the plastic tube connector back into my throat. "You know, I'm gonna stand behind him next time," she said.

The blue-eyed nurse checked the monitors. Both were walking toward the door when I made a loud grunt to get their attention.

"Do you need something else?" one of them asked. I made a writinglike gesture.

"Oh, I'll get you some paper and a pencil," she said. She walked toward the nurses' station and returned with old computer printouts.

"Here, you can use the back of these," she said. I immediately wrote, *Give me something for the pain.* She took my finger and placed it on the morphine button lying by my side.

"Push this button for morphine and this one to call us," she said. "Push it at least once every fifteen minutes." I nodded and thought, *A simple task if not in pain, but remembering what button and when was a herculean task when emotionally drained by potential death.* I quickly forgot which button to push, not that one, so I made loud grunts as I did in the past, but failed to get their attention. They walked out, leaving me alone. I felt trapped, like those lightning bugs I used to catch in mason jars on Norfolk's hot humid nights. Their energy glowed brightly until all used up.

I thought I heard my grandmother's voice ask, *Jerry, why do you live out there in California all by yourself?*

I'm not alone, Grandmother, I'm . . . established.

Boy, you don't have no kin to look after you out there, she said.

I thought I heard another familiar voice.

"Honey, wake up."

I tried opening my eyes, but like those lightning bugs, my energy was all used up.

"Honey, I'm here." Whispers continued to slowly echo through my dreams, vying for attention, as my eyelids flickered. I thought I saw Monica.

"Wake up, baby," she said. Her full lips parted with a gleaming bright smile projecting clearly, igniting happy vibes throughout my aching bedridden body.

"I'm here, baby," Monica said. She gently stroked my IV-free hand. We stared at each other, and our minds raced like hummingbirds darting about spring flowers, love glistening with each glance until a nurse entered the room and blocked my view.

"Mr. Green, it's time for your treatment," she said. A young black man followed behind her.

"Get him ready," she said. "Connect the portable oxygen bottle." He followed orders, grunting boyishly beneath his breath, as he grabbed the bottle, bent down, and connected it and asked, "Take him where?"

"To nuclear medicine," she said.

He pushed me into the people-cluttered hallway abuzz with life. They stared at my yellow, red, and green catheters, with looks of "What's wrong with him?" and "I'm glad it's not me." I closed my eyes. The gurney's wheels vibrated a pleasant-sounding melody through the catheters in my tongue. We stopped in front of a large white metal door. He rang the buzzer, and seconds morphed into minutes until the door opened.

"I'll take him from here."

"Mr. Green, do you remember me?" a man asked. He pushed me through the door.

"I met with you several times during your visits with Dr. Demanes. I'm Dan, and I'll assist the doctor with your radiation treatment," he said. Our eyes locked in familiar acknowledgment as he rolled me into a room, past a nurse with brown eyes surrounded by sweet cinnamon tones and full lips. She smiled at me.

"Are you in pain?" she asked. Her soft hand stroked my arm. I nodded yes. She pushed a button on my IV.

"Push this button every fifteen minutes for pain," she said. Her warm hand placed the button in my grip. Her eyes slowly moved out of sight, and Dan's eyes returned.

He smiled, and I stared at the ceiling while he attached my rainbow of tubes for my first treatment to a machine, called an off-loader. "Mr. Green," he said with a smile, "I'm finished connecting your catheters." His eyes retreated from view as he moved away from my multihued connections to join others behind a lead wall and started my treatment, parading radioactive isotopes down the yellow canal, then the red, and finally the green, killing good and bad cells with each trip, while shrinking my tongue from the inside out. Upon his return, he asked, "Mr. Green, how do you feel?" I gestured "OK," and he disconnected me from the off-loader. I returned and repeated the process twice a day through Thursday.

Dan opened the door and pushed me into the hallway, where I heard someone say, "Is he ready?"

"Yeah, he's all yours," Dan said. He handed me off to an orderly. *That wasn't bad*, I said to myself, feeling the morphine kick in as the orderly pushed me past scores of healthy hallway spectators on the way back to intensive care. There a nurse helped park my gurney, reconnected my lifelines, and removed me from the temporary support system.

"Remember, push this button for pain and this one to call us if you need help," she said. She left me alone. Tears welled up, but none fell; my eyes started to burn.

"Gerald, wake up," I heard someone whisper.

I awoke on Thursday, incarcerated under hell's mechanized, noisy lights. I looked and saw Monica smiling down at me, with the TV above her head still blasting OJ's pretrial mess.

How are you and how was Charles this morning? I wrote. Monica can't hide her emotions well and began sniffling.

"This was a rough morning. Charles cried a lot last night, and I didn't sleep well," she said. Monica paused for a few moments to dry her eyes, and I reached for her hand in support. I clasped it firmly and held back my tears.

"But, baby, I'm here, and we'll make it through this together," she said. Her resolve gave me strength, and I welcomed the time we would be reunited. I looked up to hear her say those words I'd learned to loathe: "I must go for now, but I'll be back after work." She leaned over and kissed me on the cheek opposite the catheters. I pushed my pain relief button and slipped back into my dreamworld.

I awoke in pain and saw my brother-in-law sitting in the guest chair looking around. Our eyes locked. Jim's voice bellowed silence away.

"Hey! Tin . . . man, I just wanted uh—wanted to come by and uh—see how you were doing. Monica told me you were outta surgery."

I grabbed my paper and wrote, *I'm glad you came by.*

"Well, fella, how you doing?"

As well as can be expected. My head hurts, I wrote.

"Is there anything I can get for you?" he asked. I nodded, just hearing Jim's deep bass tone resonated a pleasurable frequency, as if I was hearing my own voice speak. I missed the sound of my voice. Jim's deep sounds carried out into the hallway, attracting some nurses to slow down, peek inside, and smile.

Jimmy was a few years older than me; however, you couldn't tell by looking at him that he had suffered from extreme childhood eczema and asthmas. He recovered enough to play semipro football as a young adult and still works out regularly at the YMCA.

Two visitors in a couple of hours—that made me feel important. Maybe that would help my nurses treat me like one of their own, not like an orphaned patient. And if Jimmy's visit wasn't enough, my next visitor, Ms. Pierre Loving, surely made my case for normalcy.

Pierre, an attorney and friend, somehow convinced the nurses she was family. Well, she was part of our extended family, but only immediate family was admitted as visitors. Lawyers have a way of getting others to believe their story. Pierre, a tall African American woman with flaming red hair, years ago brought a smile to Uncle Emile's face by chopping vegetables for a salad. Every time she went chop-chop in her short skirt and Fry boots, her hips went boom-boom, the skirt shimmied, and Emile's eyes sparkled. Later, Emile would say, "You chop it like this." This always made Monica and me smile.

"Hi, Tinman!" she boomed. "I just wanted to come by and see how you were doing?" Her voice always sounded like she was speaking in court. She was never at a loss for words, but seeing me with tubes coming out of my face must have been difficult. She paused before asking, "Is there anything I can do for you?" I grabbed my paper and wrote.

Thanks for coming by. I'm OK considering everything that has happened.

She walked around, checking out my room, before sitting down. While she sat, a nurse dropped in and checked my instruments.

"Oh, I see you have more company, aren't you a lucky guy," she said. She checked some of the instruments and observed Pierre. I sensed Pierre was going to say something; she looked at me with one of those "don't get me started" looks. I was happy she didn't say anything because I didn't need any unnecessary drama. Pierre could give you a *Law and Order* performance. She stood up from her chair and walked toward me.

"I have to go now, and I'll check on you later," she said.

I was feeling good afterward and thought silently, *Come on, crew, come do your stuff. I'm ready, I just completed a triple dose of visitor therapy. I'm ready for the halls of stares, filled with people who dare not lock eyes with the man with the rainbow-colored tubes flowing through his cheek.*

An orderly pushed, and hallway pedestrians gawked. I caught glimpses of nasal hairs as I slipped beneath their breath on my way to my last treatment. They couldn't tell I was smiling inside, not just because of the morphine, but because I had survived my first series of cancer treatments.

"It's time," a familiar voice said.

Time for what? I thought. She came closer to my face with that trained therapeutic smile, backing up a determined look to complete her job and go home.

"It's time to check your breathing without the respirator," she said. She attached a small device to my index finger and disconnected the oxygen supply line from my trachea connector.

"Now just try and breathe normally," she said. By this time another nurse, kind of short and stubby, entered the room. She smiled like the other one did. Her body blocked my view of the nurses outside my door changing shifts at the workstation, one of the few human activities my bed-trapped body looked forward to seeing to help lessen my despair.

I sucked air down my mouth and trachea. The attendants smiled in approval.

"His breathing is great," one of the nurses said. I saw that the other one acknowledged with an up-and-down head motion. They both moved in closer from either side.

"Your lungs' oxygenation rate is excellent. We are going to take your trachea tube out," one nurse said. I wanted to celebrate, but remembered the pain associated with the last removal of the L-shaped trachea tube connector from my throat for cleaning. My hands grabbed the bedsides as a nurse placed her hands just out of my sight near my neck. I could feel her hands touching the L-shaped connector tube; my body began flinching quickly, muscle spasms everywhere, and I tightly closed my eyes, fusing my eyebrows together. I felt a quick jerk, heard a pop, and felt relief as mucus-coated air escaped. I joyously opened my eyes, took a deep breath, and felt the nurse slowly pull my feeding tube from my nose. Normal breathing and smelling, two of life's basic functions, were back—I took a deep breath, smelled my sanitized, chlorinated bed, and relished the moment when I could talk. A nurse bandaged my wound and told me I must place my fingers over my bandage to speak. I moved my fingers over my bandage.

"Thank you," I said. Hibernating facial muscles woke up.

I took in deep breaths of joy and discovered another newfound freedom, the freedom of movement and speech. I felt like my son after he pulled himself up to stand and looked around for the first time. *Isn't this great?* Charles must have thought. *I can look down at things. Oh my, what are those? Look! My feet, way down there.*

Thoughts of Charles's early life discoveries filled me, and his new experiences would become lessons for me to relearn. Now, we were at opposite ends of a conundrum. I knew how to feed myself with a fork and spoon; Charles didn't, but his body expelled waste without effort, and mine couldn't. So here I would stay until my body responded more like his.

I ate my first meal of chicken bouillon soup and Jell-O. It felt great; something warm flowed down my throat followed by a cool desert, and my stomach felt regal with its peasant portion. I sat up like a king on my throne of discomfort.

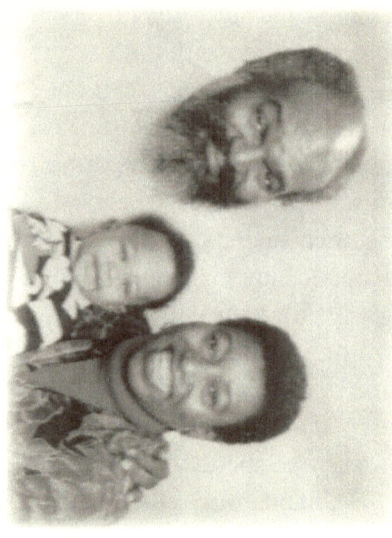

Six Months Before Treatment

During Radiation Treatment

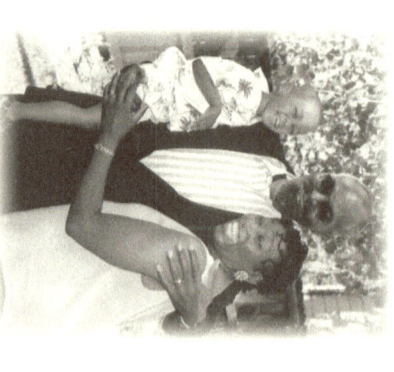

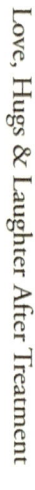

Love, Hugs & Laughter After Treatment

Deacon Mack Patillo, one of the Founders and his Family

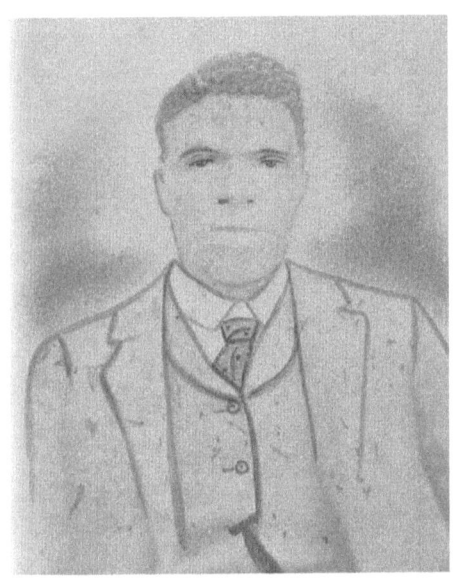

Father Mack

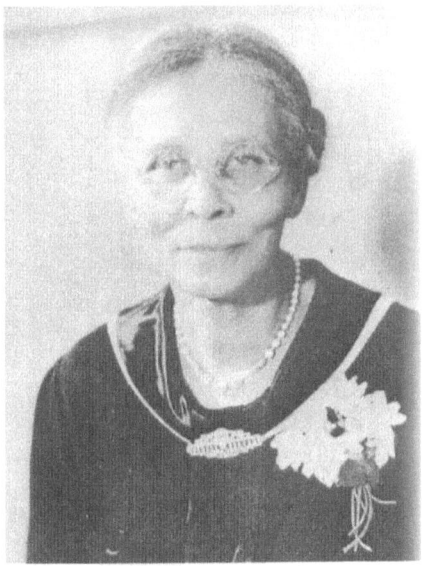

Mother Anna

O give thanks unto the Lord for he is good Ps. 107:1

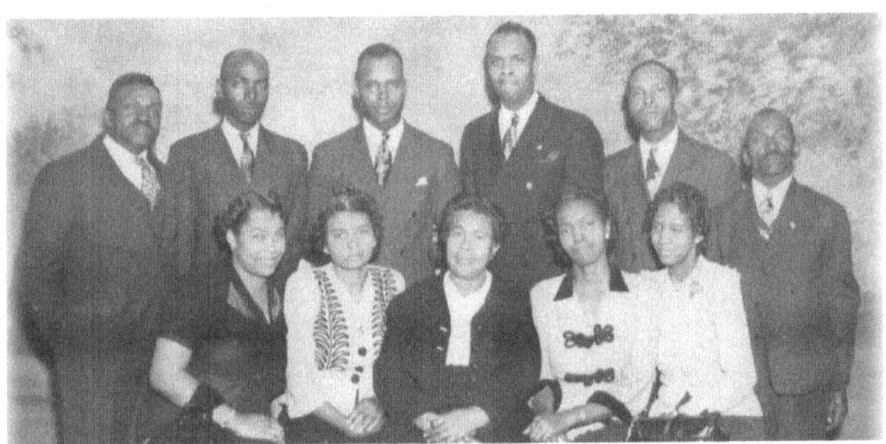

Daughters; Ann P. Jefferson, Jannette P. Jefferson, Candis P. Johnson, Mary E. Patillo, Rose P. Jefferson. Sons Charlie, Mack, Samuel, John, Corlonus, and Robert.

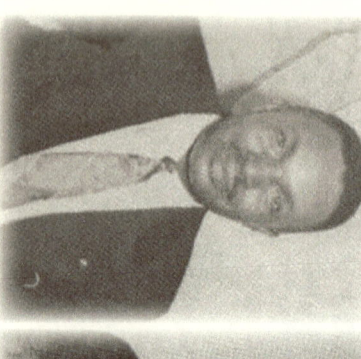

Mr. and Mrs. Patillo

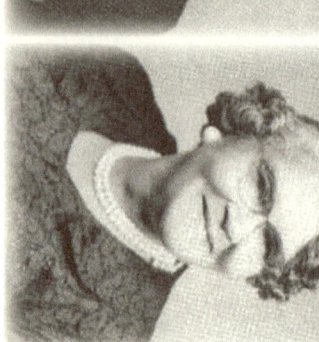

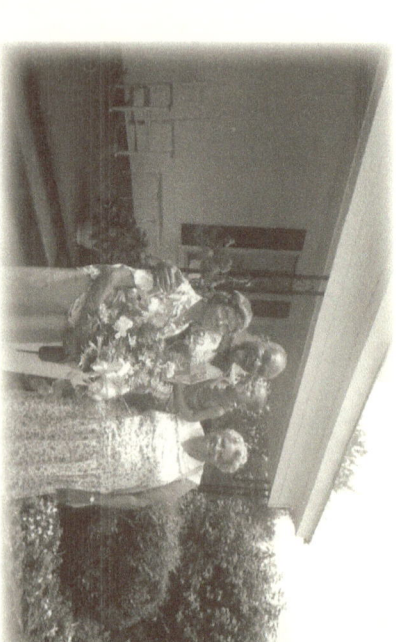

Great Aunt Mary, Charles, Mother & Me

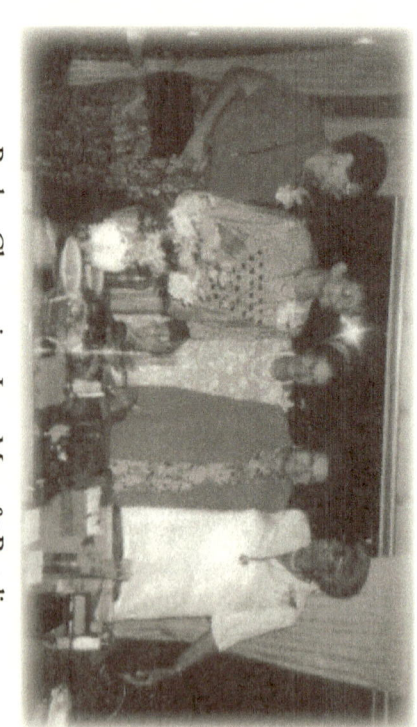

Ruthe, Clementine, Lue, Mary & Rotelia

The Patillo Sisters

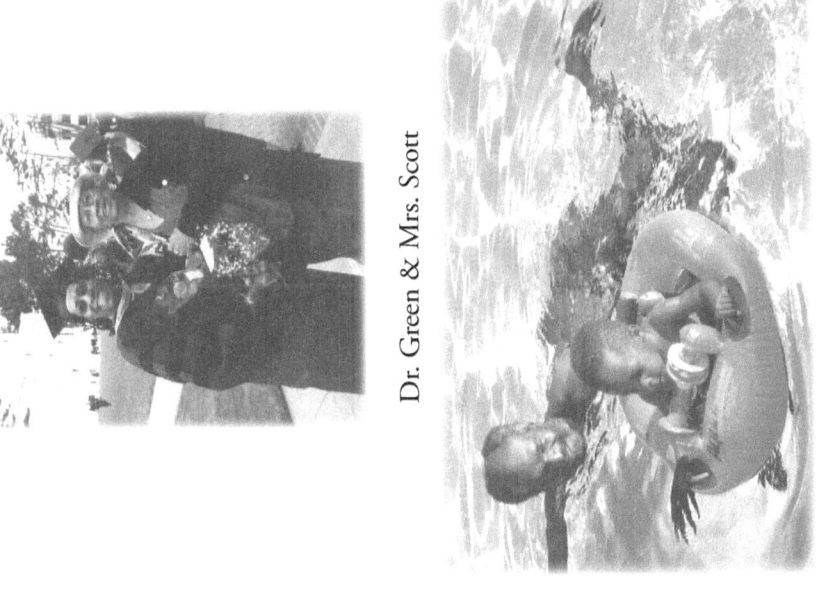

Dr. Green & Mrs. Scott

Charles and Gerald Swimming

Mother, Monica & Me

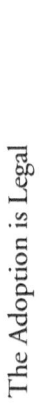

The Adoption is Legal

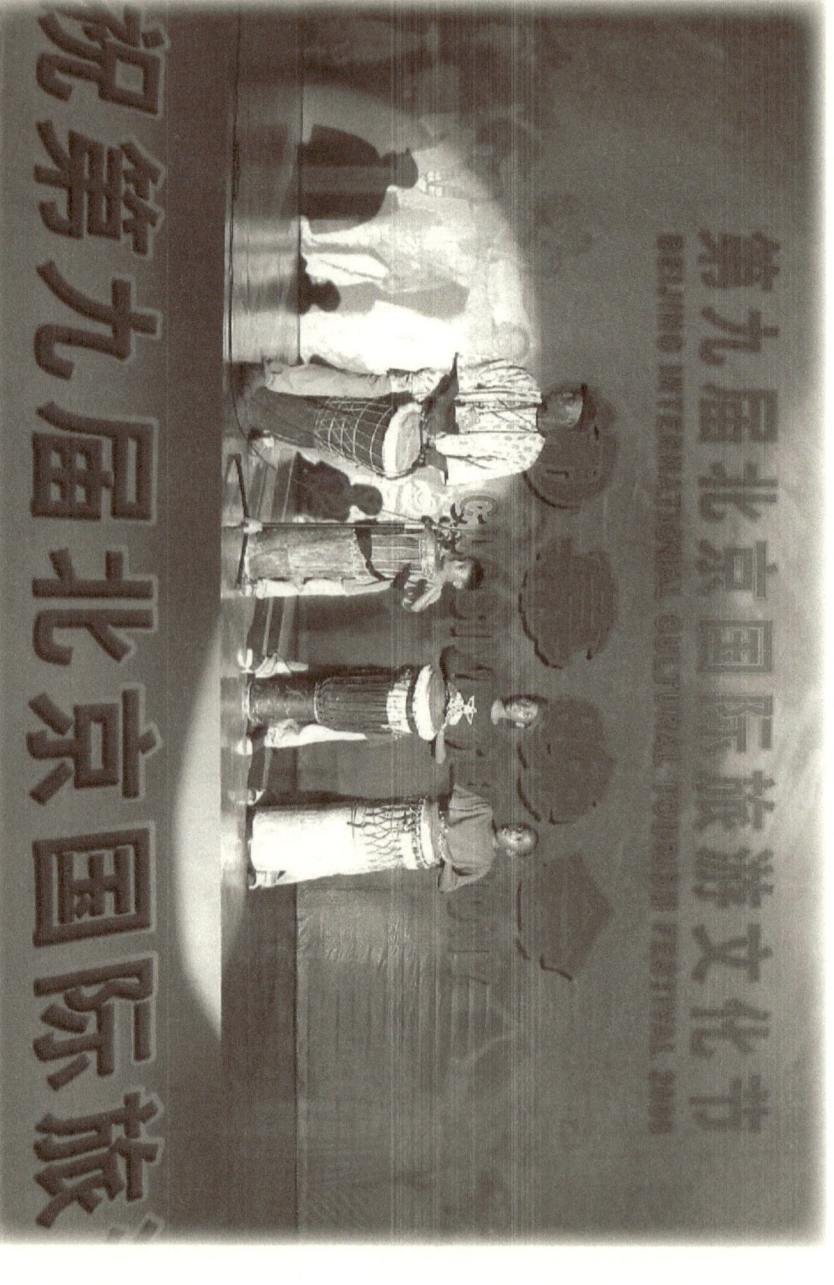

Left to right, Tacoma, Bonn, Charles, and Victor drumming in Beijing 2006

CHAPTER 9

Coming Home

MONICA PARKED IN the valet section. She exited with her body swaying to blue note tones, thumping through years of drum lessons from her father. She released transplanted New Orleans rhythmic motion, side to side, step-by-step, no music . . . just her blue note, her beat, people walking to their destinations, resonating her pleasant melodies. She walked through Friday's confectionery-scented air, eliciting intoxicated grins from strangers basking in vibrant sun, jokingly guarding the busy foyer buffer to my world without sweet air, no sun, just noisy white lights. She flashed back to the times she served the sick and poor in Denver, and she remembered having tea in San Francisco with the now-deceased Mrs. Sue Bailey Thurman and Dr. Howard Thurman, a Morehouse College—trained theology professor who taught Martin Luther King Jr. Her cherished memories vanished, and she sauntered through the automatic doors. She smiled at the security guard, and his head bobbed in rhythm to her infectious beat. She transmitted happy African gyrations with each step, and her presence pulled smiles onto lunchtime hungry faces. She ambled toward the elevator and pushed the up arrow. Her body slowed and leaned against the wall, and her eyes blinked rapidly in a failed attempt to stay open. She was asleep on her feet; the elevator doors opened, releasing a crowd that vibrated her spirit awake. She stepped across the elevator's threshold and pushed number 3 before its doors trapped her in recirculated, swishing, spicy-smelling air.

"Girl, those pork buns were great, we've got to eat there again," someone said.

"Yeah, girl, did you taste the fried rice?"

"And cheap too."

Monica stepped into a near-empty hallway. She paused for a black male attendant pushing an empty wheelchair and cried happy tears.

"It'll be OK," a passing voice whispered from behind. Monica turned, looked at the nurse with the caring eyes.

"Thank you, but I'm so happy. Sometimes I cry," she said.

"I understand. I do the same," the nurse said and handed Monica a tissue.

"Where you headed?" the nurse asked.

"Room 300," Monica said.

"That's intensive care."

"Yes, my husband is coming home today."

"God's blessings be with you," she said before embracing Monica. "Not many patients go straight home from intensive care."

Her words lifted Monica's thoughts. *Yes, we truly have the Lord's blessings.* Monica smiled; they followed the black attendant pushing the empty wheelchair toward intensive care, and she tossed her tear-filled tissue into the trash at her dirge's end.

"Excuse me," a nurse said darting from a room, startling Monica. Monica's pace quickened; she tingled with each step, and she stopped next to the nurse's island to catch her breath. She saw that the black man pushed the empty wheelchair into my room.

"Where to?" the black attendant asked. A nurse had just returned my original check-in clothes. She looked up.

"He's being released," she said.

"Released from intensive care!" said the attendant before Monica walked in.

"Oh my God, look at you," Monica said. I placed my right index and long finger over my bandaged throat and pressed it, but air seeped out around my fingers. I made squeaky sounds like a beginner saxophonist. My voice shrilled, "Hi, baby!" Her eyes gazed on my smooth black face. I pressed my throat bandage a little harder to stop the air from escaping and said, "I'm glad to see you." Her beaming face glowed when I stood. We hugged and kissed before the black attendant pushed me and the wheelchair out the door. My eyes were level with her rhythmic hips, and I watched her sashay through the hallway lunchtime crowd converting many frowns into smiles. Outside the sun kissed my face—fresh air and scented flowers welcomed me—I saw faraway green trees, and such simple pleasures began to unravel my treads of doubt that I wouldn't make a full recovery.

I enjoyed the ride through midday traffic, until my pain relief medication faded, leaving me weakened. I felt trapped in a wounded shell, and I wished the gusty sky would blow my suffering away. The gurgling noise from my stomach grew louder.

"Are you all right?" Monica asked.

"My head hurts," I said with my fingers covering my bandage. The slow ride reminded me of those painful trips on the gurney, but at least this time I was sitting and looking out the window. The car motion lulled me to sleep, and I saw Charles's little round chipmunk cheeks. I held him in my arms and felt his heartbeat. I whispered, "Daddy is home."

"Wake up, honey, we're home," Monica's distant-sounding voice said. I opened my eyes. The garage clutter robbed me of my vision of Charles.

"Do you need help getting out of the car?" Monica asked.

"I'm OK," I said. Speaking was difficult, and I didn't want to worry her about my increasing pain that drained my energy. I made an effort to stand up. Monica had reached for the balloons when she saw me slip back into the seat.

"Here, let me help you," she said. I don't know why I couldn't just accept her help. My diminished capacity clouded my judgment and tricked my body. I extended my arm, and Monica helped me out of the car and into the house. She was so excited that she carried on a conversation without me.

My first night at home, I felt something biting inside my neck.

"Help!" I said. Air escaped from around my bandage. Monica jumped.

"What's wrong, baby?" she asked.

"We got ants!"

She tossed the sheet back and hopped out of bed. I frantically waved my hands and brushed them away from my bandage. I got out of bed and stood next to a trail of ants parading across the carpet.

"Oh, Gerald, I'm sorry," she said.

"Baby, it's not your fault," I said, with my fingers over my tacky bandage. Tears trickled down her face. She helped me brush off the ants and then got rid of the remaining ones. When I woke up the next morning, Monica had taken Charles to child care and gone to work. I got up, took my medicines, and returned to bed. I later called my brother.

"Hello, David," I said over my dry lips, holding my bandage.

"Who is this?"

"David. You don't recognize me?"

"Jerry! You sound . . . different."

"Yeah, I got to press my bandage on my throat when I talk," I said. "Kind of like Coltrane playing his saxophone."

"What was that, Jerry?" David asked.

"I got to press my bandage, or air seeps out and steals my voice," I said.

"Oh . . . Does it . . . hurt?"

"Just a little," I said.

"Jerry, you sound faint."

"Oh, I forgot to press," I said, reaching for my throat.

"Don't hurt yourself. I can make out what you're saying. A little," David said. I tried licking my lips before answering, but my tongue was too dry. I sat up and drank some water.

"Thanks, I'm trying. How was Mother's gallstone surgery?"

"What was that . . . Jerry?" David asked. A little frustration flared in his voice. I pressed harder on my bandage, like Coltrane squeezing out blue notes from *A Love Supreme*. Wet air escaped between my fingers while holding my patch, slightly muting my words. "How was Mother's surgery . . . ? Da . . . Dave . . . David."

"Oh, her surgery," David answered. "Mother . . . she was a little sore for a while. But she's fine now."

"David. Did you tell her about me?" I asked.

"Oh, no. You gotta do that."

"OK, brother. I understand."

"That's right. I kept your secret, but it's on you to tell," he said.

David was right. I clung to the thought that Mother wasn't strong enough for my bad news. That was selfish of me, but David and I had agreed to spare her while she was building up strength for surgery. I hung the phone up next to the bed, closed my eyes, and prayed for sleep. But no sleep came my way.

The next day, I ate a little split pea soup, but a wad of mucus blocked me from swallowing it. My inflamed throat, once kissed by ants, heaved up the green slime on my pants and shoes. Monica turned her head. She would later champion my recovery through radiation's slow theft of my strength and spirit. Dr. Lampenfeld had designed a lead facial prophylactic shield, but it failed to prevent radiation from inflaming my tongue and throat, which forced him to stop my treatment temporarily in September. Absent strength, I rested in bed and read *My American Journey* by Colin Powell. My body shrank between each page and begged for relief, and muscle spasms stole silent slumber.

*   *   *

Weeks later, I was lying in bed looking at the ceiling when I spoke softly into the telephone.

"Hello, Mother," I said, and my eyes wandered the four corners of our bedroom while waiting for her to answer.

"Jerry, it's good to hear from you," she said. I hesitated and thought about my agreement to mislead her about my illness.

"David said you'll still sore from surgery," I said.

"Just a little, I have good days and bad days," she said in a clear voice. I listened closely to her tone, rubbed my sweating palms together, and tried to figure out if this was a good time to talk about my cancer.

"Is this a good day, Mother?" I asked in a childlike manner.

"Yes," she answered.

Without excitement I responded, "Oh."

"Jerry, you sound disappointed I feel good."

I took a long slow sip of water and licked my dry lips. "No, Mother, I'm happy for you," I said unconvincingly. Even though I didn't talk to my mother often, she could tell something was wrong.

"What's the matter, Jerry?" she asked. I searched for strength and found none. I drank more water.

"Well, Mother, I've been sick too," I said.

"You have?" she asked, and her question echoed inside me.

"I was diagnosed with tongue cancer last June," I said. I heard her gasp for air, and then the receiver went quiet.

"Mother! Are you all right?" I asked.

"Yes, Jerry, I just had to catch my breath." Her response was what I feared most, that my news would trigger a relapse. I heard her breathing slow down before the receiver slipped from my cramping left hand. I switched hands. I no longer needed to squeeze out words because the hole in my throat had closed.

"Yes, David and I thought you didn't need any more bad news before your surgery," I said.

"Jerry, thanks for thinking about me. I guess . . . you did what you thought was right," Mother said. I breathed a heavy sigh of relief. My deception seemed to have worked.

"Jerry, what kind of treatment . . . are you . . . taking?" Mother asked. Her voice sounded clear again, free of stress, and that gave me an emotional lift.

"Mother, I've completed two types of radiation therapies."

"How do you feel?" she asked.

"I'm tired most of the times. But I'm glad my treatments are over," I said.

"Me too," she said. I relaxed my grip on the telephone.

"Mother, we're planning on having Charles baptized in November. We would love for you to come."

"You are? I don't think I'll be ready to fly alone by then."

"I understand. But anyway, it's gonna be on Sunday, November 12. Maybe David will come with you?"

"OK. I'll ask him." Monica's favorite parting words, *I love you*, seeped into me.

"Good-bye, Mother—I love you."

CHAPTER 10

Reborn

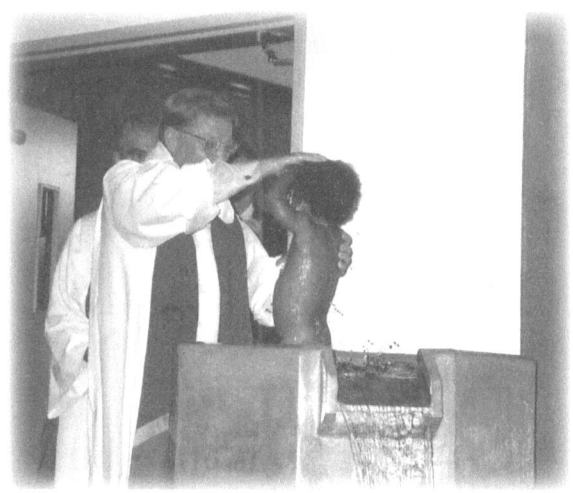

DURING THE SUMMER of 1995, Monica's faith guided plans for Charles's scheduled November baptism and tempered my summertime dirge with radiation therapy. She juggled her needs, nourished my weakened body, and took one-year-old Charles to Long Beach on her Head Start consulting job, arranging for child care before making presentations. She returned home overwhelmed by her own selfless love, caught up with demands and the potential of failing to keep up with it all. Monica stayed strong with the faith in which she was raised (thanks to her mother encouraging her father to convert to Catholicism while they were courting).

Saint Augustine's mother, an African woman who was also named Monica, similarly introduced her husband and later her adult son, Saint Augustine, to the Roman Catholic Church's baptismal waters. My mother,

Rotelia, and Monica's mother, Beatrice, continued that legacy of African women in the Diaspora leading their men to Christianity. Rotelia introduced Dad and me to the Episcopal Church. These strong black women opened masculine eyes to their need for faith. Both women—Rotelia a Protestant and Beatrice a Catholic—traveled thousands of miles to witness Charles's rebirth. My mother convinced David to fly with her. Monica's mother had suffered a heart attack a year prior, but her doctor released her in time to travel. She flew alone.

We were required to attend baptism classes in preparation for Charles's new life. At our last class, I shared my cancer experience with parents of young Christians in training. That was the first time I told anyone outside my family. Sharing my pain with others helped me reconnect to faith that I had lost in San Diego—Charles's baptism classes brought me fresh hope.

Clouds moved aside on the morning of November 12, 1995, and Charles's little hands clung to Father Roberts's white robe near his green sash. Parishioners' laughter echoed off the polished hardwood floors as they watched the resistant little bronze body dangle above the baptismal waters. Monica grabbed Charles's hand, released his fingers one at a time, before Father Roberts gained control over his wiggling body. He lowered him in the name of the Father, and everyone cheered when the baby's naked brown bottom touched the water. Then Father Roberts raised his Catholic candidate and lowered him in the name of the Son. Charles looked up, waving cheerful playtime arms and kicking water onto Father's white robe. Father Roberts elevated him on high and then lowered him in the name of the Holy Spirit. Father Roberts splashed water over heaven's new soul and anointed Charles's frizzy hair then lifted him, and parishioners' laughter converted to cheers.

I extended a white receiving blanket for my dripping son and covered his little body. I hugged him, crisscrossing my hands across his tiny back. As I rested Charles on my shoulder next to my blackened pelican-puffed throat, he looked around the church at his new family, not understanding their commitment to him, God, and their profession of faith.

Monica's green dress blended with Father Robert's sash, but her smiles exceeded his joyous blessings as she reached out to me for our son. Charles rubbed his hands on his oil-touched head and then licked them, before he focused on his mother's sound and touch. His entourage of loved ones escorted him through double doors at the back of the sanctuary into the adjacent gym, where there were tables set up under basketball hoops for families to put dry clothes on newly baptized babies. Monica and Charles's godmother dressed him in matching white African-patterned pants and top while *parrain* (the name for godfather used in New Orleans) and I stood behind them, watching. Other mommies and godmothers changed babies on tables next to Charles, with fathers and godfathers observing, before returning to the sanctuary. Young Christians dressed in white looked up at smiling faces similar to the legacy practiced by freed slaves in their metamorphic conversion to Christianity's duality—Protestants or Catholics.

Later, in our backyard, many friends gathered to help Charles celebrate his day of transition. It was an unseasonably warm November afternoon, and the sun danced on everyone's faces until twilight's chill. I watched them eat and remembered the fresh smell of Grandmother's dinner rolls rising atop her refrigerator. My hunger pains grew, but the thought of tasteless food robbed my desire to eat, like Sisyphus's curse.

I later went to bed, but sleep failed to rescue me from my anxiety and depression. I thought I heard Rahsaan Roland Kirk singing "Bright Moments" and playing multiple saxophones and a nose flute, with air I gasped for. That memory took me back in time, and I saw him playing New Orleans blues to the Berkeley crowd. The night he followed the tambourine man offstage singing "Volunteered Slavery" while playing his instruments. The club sang, "Volunteered slavery . . . good God, you gotta be free . . . volunteered slavery . . ." as we followed the blind pied piper onto Tenth and University. We sang and danced behind him up to San Pablo Avenue and then returned to the smoke-filled club. The performance brought me bright moments.

I moistened my dry, chapped lips like I was going to play a saxophone, and sleep came.

*   *   *

Dr. Watson's dazzling smile entered the examination room decorated with a painting of a Masai warrior whose deep piercing eyes helped me lower my guard.

"Gerald, how are you feeling today?" he asked.

"Doctor, my mouth hurts . . . and I can't eat . . . much," I said. My eyes were still fixed on the proud dark-skin warrior in the painting. I wondered what ills threatened him and wept silently, thinking about my uncertainty. I felt helpless and alone. I needed the Masai's courage.

"Now where does it hurt?"

"My tongue . . . it hurts inside."

"Gerald, what are you taking for the pain?"

"Tylenol with codeine," I said, "but it doesn't work all of the time."

"You gotta take it even if you don't feel any pain. The key to pain management is pain prevention," he said before leaning over and pressing on my shoulders near the yoke of my neck.

"Does this hurt?" he asked.

"No," I said. He pressed another spot and repeated the question. I gave him the same answer—no.

"I see you're still losing weight," Dr. Watson said.

"Yeah, it's hard to eat when you can't taste anything," I said.

"Take a deep breath," he said. I jumped when he placed his cold stethoscope on my back.

"Hold it. OK, relax."

Air rushed out of my mucus-clogged throat. I reached for my water bottle, took a sip, and licked my lips. Dr. Watson wrote something in my chart and then looked up from his round swivel stool.

"Gerald, you must stop losing weight. You know, Dr. Demanes is thinking about ordering you a feeding tube," he said.

I looked at him in disbelief. My eyes sank backward. Mentally, I focused on the sculptured African woman's head with tight knotlike braids that I had seen. Her bronze smile brought me calm, and I relaxed my grip on the side of the examination bed.

"Gerald, can't you eat something, like mashed potatoes and gravy?" he asked.

"I tried eating split pea soup, but I couldn't keep it down."

"You can't continue losing weight if you want to heal," he said.

"What can I do?" I asked.

"How about mixing ice cream with your Ensure?"

"Yeah, that sounds good."

He wrote in my chart again, then took a small pad out of his pocket.

"Here, Gerald, just in case you need more pain medicine," he said.

"Thanks, Dr. Watson," I said, hoping that the ice cream and Ensure would save me from forced feeding. I placed my hands on my knees and lowered my head toward the floor.

"I have another problem," I said.

"What kind of problem?" he asked.

"I ran out of sick leave."

"Don't you have long-term disability insurance?"

"Yeah, but it won't make me whole," I said. Dr. Watson stopped walking toward the door and looked back at me. Our eyes connected.

"What do you think about me going back to work?" I asked.

"Gerald, what about your pain?" he asked. I knew he was right about my pain and nervously shifted my eyes back and forward to avoid further contact. "I talked to my supervisor yesterday about working from home," I said. "He said I could train on a software called SAP from my home computer."

"How many hours a day?" Dr. Watson asked.

"As many as I can do, at my own pace," I said. Dr. Watson frowned.

"That's not a good idea!" he said.

"But my family needs the money."

"Gerald, you're gonna have to decide whether your health is more important than money."

"I understand what you're saying, but I need to return to work," I said.

"OK, but I want to see you in three weeks," Dr. Watson said.

Three weeks later, I told Dr. Watson I felt better, which was a lie, and not my first one either. I resorted to deceit in my pursuit of work. Dr. Watson had grown up listening to his father's patients' casual deception, and he wasn't convinced.

I returned to a forty-hour workweek. I worked from January 1996 to the middle of February before pain made work unbearable.

The Man in the Blue Chamber

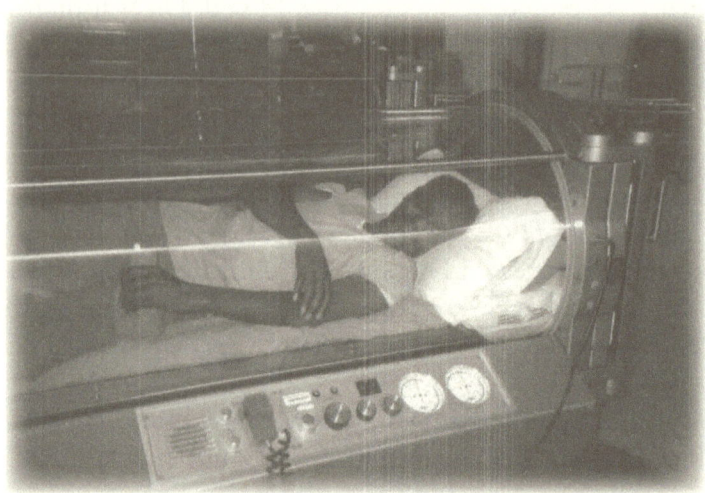

IN THE SPRING of 1996, fifteen pairs of hands took turns feeling my tongue at the tumor board, where Dr. Michael Kaplan was the lead oncologist. Unlike the other doctors, he didn't believe my cancer had metastasized. But in his matter-of-fact tone, he explained if it was cancer, then his surgical team would have to reconstruct my jawbone using a small bone from my lower leg and remove a portion of my tongue, before they woke me from the biopsy procedure.

"You're lucky, it's just radiation necrosis. Your pain comes from internal scarring, a byproduct of radiation therapy," Dr. Kaplan said afterward. Happy tears rolled down the right side of my burned-black face. A smile larger than his small frame illuminated the room, and from that moment on, Monica and I looked forward to his medical counsel. I would later receive four weeks of ninety minutes per day hyperbaric oxygen therapy sessions for pain relief.

At my first treatment for pain, a technician greeted me with a Southern drawl. "Howdy. Are you ready?" he asked. His voice reminded me of the not-so-good old boys from my 1950s childhood. My anxiety soared when he opened what looked like a blue-frame iron lung with a submarine hatch—like cover.

"Yes, I'm ready," I replied, but I lied (mentally I wasn't prepared).

"Are you claustrophobic?" he asked, before pulling out a small flat gurney bed from the blue healing chamber.

"No." I said.

"Here, take this. It'll relax you," he said in his gatekeeper's voice. "You should feel your ears . . . tightening." The pressure increased, and the glass walls hugged me tight like slaves packed in the hull of a ship. My eyes flickered. I looked up at the television through the convex glass, and the background music slowly relaxed me. I fell asleep and recalled one of my favorite childhood memories of skipping down gravel-covered Workwood Road in Chesapeake Gardens with cousins to Grandmother's house. It was when I felt most secure—kicking stones in one of Norfolk's 1950s segregated communities. I remembered looking up at them as they teased me while we walked. They constantly tried to avoid swarms of gnats that I simply walked under. I wanted to keep up with them, but their legs were almost as long as I was tall. They would run off and leave me alone to skip to Grandmother's house. Sometimes when the weak part of my shoes hit sharp-edged stones not worn down by cars, I jumped because those sharp hot stones cut my foot. I felt relieved upon arriving at Grandmother's house because she had a smooth concrete walkway from the street to her front door, flanked on both sides by roses, which I saw from their bottoms. Usually, I ran up to the porch, next to those thorny sweet-smelling giant roses abuzz with big black bumblebees. Best of all was opening the storm door with the capital *P*, which stood for Patillo, before entering a little kid's paradise. Grandmother's living room had three tables with lots of whatnot figurines for a kid to play with, although her rule was, "Don't touch." All the grandkids played with the brightly painted opaque figurines, and Grandmother spanked those she caught. Playing with them was fun, and what I remembered most about those whatnots was licking their sour-tasting bottoms; it must have been the lead—a taste I hope Charles never experiences.

Charles and I would, years later, return to Workwood Road on the Fourth of July to celebrate colored people's fiftieth anniversary of home ownership in Chesapeake Gardens's enclave protection from white Southern brutality.

My old haven, the woods and marsh, had been replaced with highways and sound walls that failed to keep the neighborhood quiet. Many houses still boasted green front yards full of roses and bumblebees; however, 860 Workwood Road no longer had a capital *P*. Mother and her sisters had sold the house. And like rhythmic singing cicadas rising from the ground to feed, we sampled cuisines in front yards. I later saw Charles sitting with a group of children on the grass listening attentively in a crisscross applesauce position that he hated in kindergarten. An elder called out names of the founding families of Workwood Road from a quilt. Tears and sweat clung to my cheeks as she read, "Charlie and Cornelia Patillo." I heard them whisper, "Present." In time, many families ventured from this safe harbor in pursuit of the American dream, only to live through decades of turbulent transition. Some have returned.

*   *   *

My eyes flickered, and the chamber shrank. I recalled a haunting high school memory of a moonless rainy night when I drove our family car down a rural two-lane road swallowed up by pine trees on either side. A friend and I were returning from a party, and I collided with another car traveling in the opposite direction. We woke up underneath the Ford facedown in cold Maryland mud. The ambulance driver and police had rolled our semiconscious bodies under the car, thinking we were safer there. An ambulance took away white passengers. We waited for hours before a second ambulance came and took us to the naval hospital. Thoughts of seeing my father after wrecking the family car on the way home from an unauthorized dance eclipsed my pain.

This type of flashback to second-class medical treatment compromised my trust in doctors. The technician and I were about the same age, and his accent suggested he too grew up in a segregated America, similar to my experiences in the mid-'60s when I integrated a Maryland high school. Feeling the impact of the pill, I drifted down those hated hallways where many students relentlessly peppered me with "nigger, go home." I fought their sickness by focusing on achieving academic excellence, to the dismay of some of my teachers who stood behind me while I took their tests.

I shuddered at the thought of looking up and seeing one of them standing over me. I twitched and bumped my head on the glass. A vision of Monica's left hand resting on a mound of green seedless grapes nestled

GERALD GREEN

in her lap next to a book returned. She methodically alternated munching grapes and reading. She avoided looking at empty scenery populated with disappearing highway markers and swallowed. I stared at cars vanishing into radiant heat waves on the horizon as I drove.

"Do we have anything cool to drink?" I asked.

"What was that?"

"Do we have any cool drinks?"

"Wouldja like water, juice, or a soda?"

"Give me a Coke."

Monica reached into the small cooler next to the door. She opened the can, while protecting her manicured fingernails, and wrapped a napkin around its base. I reached toward her red-tipped and pink-striped fingertips. Our hands met above the stick shift, where she gave me the sweating can. I took a long sip then wedged it between my legs, never breaking my concentration from the highway.

"What're you reading?" I asked.

"An anthology of poetry from *American Negro Poetry*," she said. Cool air danced around her face.

"Would you like to hear one?" she asked.

"Sure."

She turned through a few pages before stopping and cleared her throat.

> Because I had loved so deeply,
> Because I had loved so long,
> God in His great compassion
> Gave me the gift of song.

Monica licked her lips, looked at me, and then continued:

> Because I have loved so vainly,
> And sung with such faltering breath,
> The Master, in infinite mercy,
> Offers the boon of death.

The smooth vibration of the vintage 164E Volvo lulled her to sleep, and I reached for grapes near her thighs engulfed in the tan leather seat. She awoke, staring at me—the man who took her grocery shopping and gave her Saturday rides from Oakland to the San Francisco African American

Cultural Society (SFAACS). She was the executive director of the SFAACS, and I was becoming more than a volunteer worker.

I slowed for the freeway exit. We saw hundreds of black-and-white heifers grazing in a field. Diesel fumes punctuated with the smell of cow manure smothered patrons standing on scorching concrete at the gas station's pumps. My short-sleeve shirt clung to my dripping body. Monica's knitted dress kept her cool, but she jumped when she returned and sat on the sunbaked leather seat. I started the car, turned the air conditioner up, and drove back to Interstate 5 South. Monica reclined her seat, picked up her book, and read me another poem.

The poem is by Paul Laurence Dunbar, from *Lyrics of Sunshine and Shadow*, published 1905.

*   *   *

I emerged from the blue chamber with Monica in my heart. I wore thin light blue static-proof clothing with matching booties to reduce the potential of a spark and fire while I was inside the chamber's oxygen environment. The technician helped me stand on weak knees, and I meandered across the cold floor into the changing room. My tongue's pain ebbed at the end of my first treatment. Monica drove home. As I sat in the passenger seat, the lingering effect of the blue chamber continued to bring back old memories. I recalled how love had compromised our resolve not to socialize at the SFAACS while we worked and how we spent our honeymoon on Paradise Island in the Bahamas. I remembered Monica wanted a house with lots of light and a backyard where we could play badminton. I wanted a swimming pool. We found our dream house in the Oakland Hills, a 1960s California ranch. It had a cathedral ceiling in the living room. Sunlight streamed through its five wooden-framed windowpanes that stretched from the floor to the ceiling and created a haven for plants. It had a park-size backyard complete with a kidney-shaped swimming pool and even a pool house.

Charles was born on June 6, 1994. Abandoned by his biological father, his mother decided she couldn't raise a baby alone. Her faith that Monica and I would give her newborn a better home led us to become first-time parents though we were both in our midforties. Then, a year after Charles's birth, I was diagnosed with tongue cancer. I received extensive radiation therapy and endured the blue chamber for relief from radiation's killing field within my tongue. His preschool teachers and other parents thought we were grandparents. That age differential forced us to exercise daily. We walked in open space within an eyeshot from our backyard, and occasionally, an off-leash dog startled Charles. One evening, we sat with him in front of the fireplace, and the red glow reflected off Monica's smile as she read aloud a children's book about adoption. His big brown eyes wandered before his attention focused on the fire. He didn't seem to care about the animal characters in the story. Monica gave me a perplexed look and then told him that just like Fuzzy Bear, he was adopted.

"I would have carried that secret to my grave," my mother told me later. Her forceful voice reminded me of arguments she had with Dad when he returned home after six months at sea. He eventually replaced us with golf, and my relationship with him all but ended after he deserted Mother for a mistress and two sons in the Philippines. He later retired from the navy, moved back to Oklahoma all alone, and married a woman not much older than me.

Hesitantly, I had called him when I became ill, but neither of us shared the small talk gene. Our words got lost over the telephone line, and cramps rolled up my neck. My hands sweated, and I stammered, "I was diagnosed with cancer."

"You were?" he said. "I'm sorry to hear that. How're you doing?"

"I'm OK," I said.

"How's that boy of yours?" he asked.

"Fine," I said with pride. "We were fortunate that we were able to adopt him as an infant."

"Oh." My unease diminished the more we talked, but the tone of his voice hung in my ear.

"Yeah, and when we told him he was adopted, he just continued to play," I said. That was the longest we had talked in years, without me getting upset about something—until . . .

"Jerry, I adopted you," he said. I dropped the phone.

"You did?"

"I thought your mother told you."

My wounded heart quickened, and silent tears tumbled into a world I once knew. Later, when I came across a photo of my deceased biological father, I carefully examined his face. What traits had I inherited, I wondered. Was one of them desertion?

*   *   *

At the end of my treatment, I could still feel radiation's barbed fingers constricting around frayed nerves inside my tongue when I swallowed water—my body melted away, exposing my exhausted muscles. I was too weak to play with Charles. I was incarcerated in a starving body, tormented by food's aroma, and grew jealous watching Monica eat. Doctors wanted me to consume at least a six-pack of Ensure Plus a day, but my hibernating taste buds made that task impossible. I camouflaged the Ensure with French vanilla ice cream and slurped down a half gallon every three days, producing large amounts of gas that percolated in my loose bowels. Sometimes errant farts chased me into the bathroom before I could get relief. Timing was everything.

I replaced Ensure with seasoned split pea soup and had pancakes drenched with butter and syrup, with milk on the side for breakfast. I started walking on the treadmill for five minutes, then ten, and twenty minutes, to combat pounds invading my once-weakened body. Monica warned me about my night purchases, but I continued to cruise neighborhood grocery stores in search of a food fix.

Eighteen months later, I was diagnosed with neck cancer and underwent surgery a week before Christmas. Monica's smile and Charles's chipmunk cheeks and chubby-arm hugs warmed my heart. Painkillers allowed me to enjoy the moment.

CHAPTER 12

Family Commitment

A SMALL DUCKLING swam alone on placid Lake Merritt, with his breast leaning forward in the thick brackish water. A wake formed in the shape of a V behind him, and a group of ducks flew above. They quacked and jousted into a wedge pattern. The duckling's innate potential to travel in such patterns strengthens his chances of keeping up with his family when it comes time to migrate.

Monica and I introduced baby Charles to Kwanzaa—his survival V pattern. We toiled daily to maintain our home grounded in *nguzo saba*, the seven principles of Kwanzaa, as we prepared our angel for his flight in a turbulent world that sees little black boys as an ugly gateway to manhood, not worthy of freedom. We pumped him full of *nia* (purpose) and *imani* (faith), in hopes a shield of Teflon would protect him from constant assault by a society blind to his humanity. We clothed him in *kujihagulia* (self-determination) as we pushed him further out on branches of his decisions until his wings either spread like the giant raptor that catches a gust of wind and carries him away on prosperity's breeze or like a homing pigeon that returns him home to surrogate parents, who would in turn pray that he accomplishes *ujima* (collective work and responsibility). We prayed that he would return to Workwood Road and Saint Paschal Church, in time to celebrate their respective one hundredth anniversaries. Maybe by then, both communities will reflect America's hue; and God will have touched homes with his blessings of *umoja* (unity) of faith, family, and friends.

I tried to hide my illness from Charles, but as he grew, my neck scar became a constant reminder. He didn't understand that he was one of the lucky ones. At least he had a father who loved him daily. I prayed that black sperm donors will retrieve their offspring from urban pain. Wake up, black men; breathe in *kuumba* (creativity) to improve our community's quality of life while practicing *ujamaa* (cooperative economics). We must rise together in victory over dysfunction and despair.

∗　　∗　　∗

David and I listened to the minister eulogize Dad into sainthood from the back of the surprisingly integrated church. We had forgotten about his religious conversion after he abandoned our mother, and his new church community only knew him as a loving husband and father of two daughters, not a man with unfilled commitments. At Dad's funeral, I met his grandson from his first wife, my mother was his second—a fact Dad hid from me and my brothers and sisters. Dad's grandson told me how much he loved playing golf with his grandfather. I couldn't help but recall how cheated I felt when Dad returned home from six months at sea and left us to play golf, but to listen to his grandson's joy and witness his love for his wife and children gave me pause to look at Dad through a different set of lenses, the same lens set I now use to observe doctors.

Although my pain continues, joy flourishes with simple pleasures like tasting good food and talking to family and friends—I'm privileged with breath and life's experiences that I may offer to those caught in cancer's grip. I'm living proof that time heals emotional and physical scars. My first scar is hidden within my tongue, where external gamma-beam treatment killed the tumor, but left scar tissue where it once thrived. This invisible scar sapped my life's pleasure. Two years after tongue cancer, I washed my face and smiled in the mirror at the new scar on my neck, a constant reminder of my second cancer surgery. It is the source of great pleasure and sometimes throbs. I get joy from looking at it and think of the consequence of not having a metastasized tumor discovered. What's a little daily pain in exchange for years of life? I've been told an amputee has phantom pains. Who am I to complain about background soreness on a body part that still functions?

Between the two scars, which one would I trade in? Neither. I have grown with these pains; they are a part of who I am. To trade them in would be to deny me—a survivor—cancer free and ready for life.

A life filled of joy and love of family,
A life that gives back to my community,
A life struggling to be the best father,
A life with love,
A life with Monica,
A life with dancing memories,
A life with scars, the scars that blessed me with another day!

EPILOGUE

I DISCOVERED A few weeks prior to our 2008 summer vacation that my prostate-specific antigen (PSA) score had jumped from 2.2 to 3.15. A PSA test is a common way to screen for prostate cancer. Although it was within the lab report's good reference range from 0.0 to 4.0, two things stuck in my mind. First, my previous PSA scores had moved up in small increments, and this one was up almost an entire point. And second, my neighbor who has survived prostate cancer for over nine years had told me many times when a black man's PSA score goes over 2.5, he should be concerned. Well, I was, but not enough to have a biopsy before my vacation.

We arrived in Raleigh, North Carolina, two days before the reunion. Charles, now fourteen, spent most of the time with his teenage cousins playing video games; and Monica and I settled into a quiet routine of morning walks. On Friday, the first day of the reunion, I greeted family members arriving for check-in. Relatives from all five Patillo sisters came, and two of the three surviving sisters were present. Charles and his cousins splashed in the swimming pool while adults sipped refreshing drinks. We looked at old pictures and videos from previous reunions that sparked intense dialogue about who remembered what. Everyone enjoyed the home-cooked and catered cuisine on Saturday; and we played bid whist, dominoes, and other board games. Budding family poets read on Sunday, the last day of the reunion, and we said blessing for the deceased. Everyone clung to precious memories, and I remembered how Mother thought my brothers and I were sick if we didn't eat seconds at dinner. And now we struggle to maintain healthy weight.

As we drove away from the reunion, sheets of rain flushed away views of trees' green canopies, and darkening clouds hid daylight. The car hydroplaned, and lightning lit up the sky, but that didn't faze Charles. He stayed glued to his electronic game's flashing screen. Monica's voice crackled, and I pulled off the road. Unlike our first trip, we had no grapes to share as rain pelted the car. Our breath fogged the windows, and a crescendo of thunderclaps finally scared Charles. He dropped his toy.

Eventually, the sun came out and bake dried sides of trees whose inner growth rings had witnessed runaway slaves escaping through the thicket. Unfortunately, some were trapped, returned, and hung from local branches. My great-grandfather survived that American tragedy and pooled his resources with several families to purchase land, after the Civil War, on which they built the Chapel on the Hill Baptist Church. He and his descendants, and members of those other families, are buried adjacent to the building; and my mother rests a few rows down a gentle slope from them, a stone's throw from creeks that once nourished crops. Charles, Monica, and I held hands, bowed our heads, and said a prayer at her grave; and fond childhood memories visited me.

Every summer, Mother would bring me to a big white house, surrounded by corn and tobacco, where her father grew up with his ten brothers and sisters, about a mile down a dusty road from the church. The elders would get up before dawn, eat a big breakfast, and go to work, many in the fields. I shared breakfast with them, but instead of working, I chased chickens and ran through the fields' red soil. Mother's thin lips would smile at me while we swung in the porch swing on those cool evenings drinking fresh lemonade.

None of the circuitous, mazelike dirt roads had names then, but Mother navigated them with ease. Now they are paved, and many carry her relatives' last names. During a recent visit, one of her cousins saw the resemblance in my face. "That's Rotelia's boy," she said. Those words made me feel loved. I want that kind of love for Charles too.

Unfortunately, Monica had to fly back to Oakland and work a couple of weeks before returning to Raleigh for her cousin's daughter's wedding. Charles went to hang out with my sister, LeAnn. She had recently purchased a beautiful two-story 1960s-type house in the once-white community of Bowie, Maryland, where all her adjacent streets started with the letter A. It was bigger than the 1950s house in Chesapeake Gardens, Virginia, where she grew up without Dad. Mother loved LeAnn and Crystal, but she didn't smother them with food. Instead, she showered them with compassion, a compassion LeAnn shares with foster-care children with special needs; and Crystal applies it to her medical-related work. Mother helped raise LeAnn's children, and when I see her youngest daughter, I'm reminded of Mother's love for reading. I'm thirteen years older than LeAnn; however, her daughters are older than Charles, and hopefully they will share Mother's spirit with him.

While Charles basked in cousin and aunt heaven, I flew to Chicago. During my first trip years ago, I got lost near dismal-looking high-rise tenement projects. I felt vulnerable then and afraid to ask strangers for directions. No high-rise projects cluttering the skyline this time, and I enjoyed listening to the navigation system's feminine voice direct me around town. I visited the DuSable Museum and strolled through the exhibit Red, White, Blue & Black: A History of Blacks in the Armed Services, which included Soul Soldiers: African Americans and the Vietnam Era. Looking at the display brought back memories of Foe-head's death, and I cried—like I did years ago when I saw his name on the Vietnam Veterans Memorial Wall. A couple days later, I sat in the Second Baptist Church of Detroit's dim-lit basement and listened to a gray-haired dreadlocked woman passionately share her church's role in the Underground Railroad. I felt her words echo off the backs of those nocturnal travelers, who hid in wagons hauling manure to avoid capture—a stench that became their freedom smell. I drew strength from their flight and the courage of my ancestors, who built farming communities among the hangman's noose.

Charles and I took a day trip to the International Spy Museum in Washington DC. We went on maneuvers with a museum operative to retrieve a nuclear trigger from a terrorist. Charles and I worked together to break spy codes and then became trapped in an elevator that shook violently. He grabbed my arm when the lights went out. We toured exhibits on ancient military spies and women spies in Civil War. Charles complained, "This is boring," until he saw James Bond's Aston Martin. We flew to Raleigh the next day, rented a car, and drove to Atlanta, where we saw old civil rights film clippings at the Martin Luther King Center. We visited cousins and saw other sites before rejoining Monica in Raleigh for the wedding.

*   *   *

Déjà vu, I heard click, click.

The doctor removed his staple gun—like instrument from my hemorrhaging rectum. I whimpered like a wounded animal, and my muffled cries escaped from the tiny room. He carefully placed the sample on the tray before reloading a fresh needle and reinserting.

Click, click: he snatched another piece of my prostate.

At sixty, I have survived tongue and neck cancer for fourteen years with no guarantees, just daily opportunities to share love. Now prostate cancer has provided yet another thread to weave into my life's fabric.

Isn't the third time a charm?

Support Data

Dr. Watson helped me develop the numerical values for pain description, and I used song titles and phrases to lighten it up. I created the values for mental and physical condition and comfort eating and combined them into a rating system I called the state of being (SOB) with a maximum value of 15.

Pain Description

Rating	Pain Description	Required
-10	Maximum	Morphine
-9	A Real Mother for You	Morphine
-8	It Hurt So Bad	Duraesic 100 mcg/hr. patch and morphine sulfate
-7	It Hurt So Bad	Duraesic 50 mcg/hr. patch and Tylenol with codeine liq.
-6	It Hurt So Bad	Duraesic 50 mcg/hr. patch
-5	I Can't Stand It	Dilaudid pill 25 mcg/ hr. patch after W 159
-4	A Major Pain	Tylenol with codeine pill
-3	A Real Pain in the Butt (Mouth)	Tylenol with codeine liq. / morphine sulfate after W 62 / aspirin after W 141
-2	Tingles and Burns	Various rinses
-1	Wired Sensations	Cold water / focus on external
0	None	Nothing

Mental and Physical Condition

Rating	Description	Required and/or Comments
1	I Could Kick the Bed Apart	Ativan
2	Up Tight	Tylenol
3	I Can't Get No Satisfaction	Rest in bed
4	Sleepless in Seattle	Relaxation / some reading and writing
5	O Lord, Let Me Rest	Relaxation, able to read and write more
6	I'm Starting to Feel All Right	Enjoy simple pleasure of my son's smile, and read and write more

7	Things Are Looking Better	Able to relax and accomplish 1-2 hour task
8	It's All Right	Enjoy basic pleasures and accomplish 3-6 hour task
9	I'm Moving On Up	Enjoy most pleasures and accomplish 7-9 hour task
10	I've Got It	Everything is working just great

Comfort Eating

Rating	Description	Comments
-5	Mouth hurts / consumed only (@)	Hospital feeding
-4	Mouth hurts / consumed only (@)	Water and 1 can of Ensure Plus/day (#)
-3	Mouth hurts/ consumed only (@)	Water and 2-3 cans of Ensure Plus w/ ice cream/day (#!)
-2	Discomfort eating (@)	4+ cans of Ensure Plus w/ ice cream/ day minimum taste/eating
-1	Some discomfort eating (@)	Some taste and eating foods Ensure Plus w/ ice cream
0	Minimum discomfort eating	Taste at 95% eating variety of foods
1	Starting to enjoy eating	Start using upper and lower partial
2	Enjoying eating more	Selection of foods improving
3	Enjoying eating more	Selection of foods improving
4	Enjoying eating more	Selection of food at 90% of normal
5	Eating most foods	Selection and taste at 100% of normal

Note: This symbol @ means dry mouth. This symbol # means food had no taste. This symbol ! means I could taste some sweets.

The First Sixty-Seven Weeks

Weeks	1	2	3	4	5	6	7	8	9	10	11	12	13	14	15	16	17	18	19	20	21	22	23	24	25
Pain description	0	0	0	0	0	0	0	0	0	0	0	0	0	0	0	0	0	0	0	0	0	0	0	-2	-2
Mental and physical condition	10	10	10	10	10	10	10	10	10	10	10	10	10	10	10	10	10	10	10	10	10	10	10	10	10
Comfort eating	5	5	5	5	5	5	5	5	5	5	5	5	5	5	5	5	5	5	5	5	5	5	5	4	4
Weekly total	15	15	15	15	15	15	15	15	15	15	15	15	15	15	15	15	15	15	15	15	15	15	15	12	12

Weeks	26	27	28	29	30	31	32	33	34	35	36	37	38	39	40	41	42	43	44	45	46	47	48	49	50
Pain description	-2	-2	-2	-3	-3	-3	-10	-5	-5	-5	-4	-4	-4	-4	-4	-4	-4	-4	-4	-3	-3	-3	-3	-2	-2
Mental and physical condition	10	10	7	7	8	8	1	3	3	4	4	4	3	4	4	4	5	5	5	6	6	6	7	7	8
Comfort eating	4	4	4	5	5	5	-5	-1	-1	-1	-4	-4	-4	-4	-3	-3	-2	-2	-2	-2	-2	-2	-2	-2	-1
Weekly total	12	12	9	9	10	10	-14	-3	-3	-2	-4	-4	-5	-4	-3	-3	-1	-1	-1	1	1	1	2	3	5

Weeks	51	52	53	54	55	56	57	58	59	60	61	62	63	64	65	66	67
Pain description	-2	-2	-1	-1	-1	-1	-1	-3	-4	-6	-9	-8	-8	-8	-8	-8	-8
Mental and physical condition	8	8	8	8	9	9	8	8	7	6	4	4	4	4	4	4	4
Comfort eating	-1	-1	0	0	0	0	0	-1	-1	-3	-3	-3	-2	-2	-2	-2	-2
Weekly total	5	5	7	7	8	8	7	4	2	-3	-8	-7	-6	-6	-6	-6	-6

Graph of the state of being for the first sixty-seven weeks

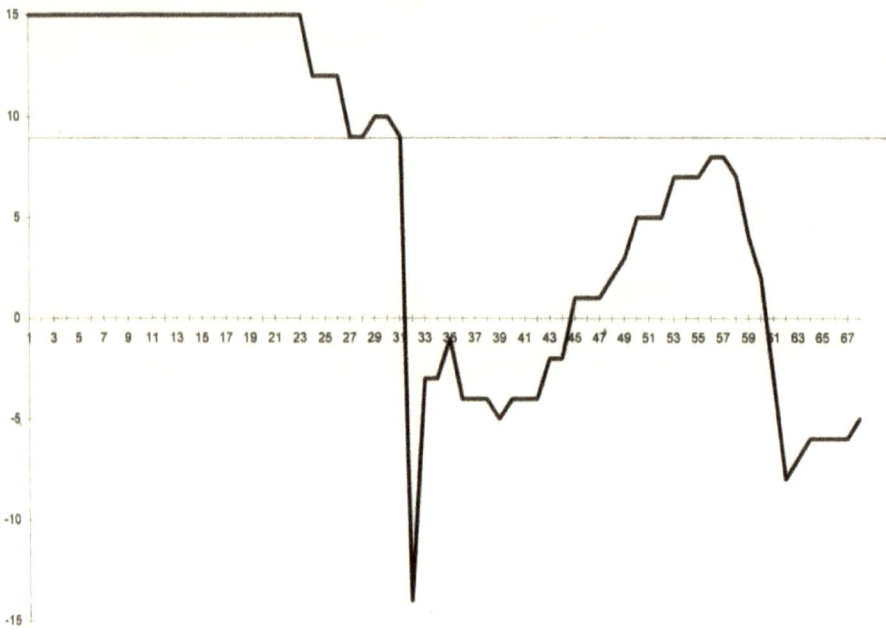

The straight line equals a value of 9 and decreasing numerically below it represents life with increasing pain.

Gerald Green
10425 Greenview Dr.
Oakland, CA 94605

November 24, 1995

Retired General Colin Powell
Mc Lean, VA 22101

Dear Colin,

We are an African American Family with a seventeen month old son. Our family's future dramatically changed on June 30, 1995, when I was diagnosed with carcinoma of the tongue. Because of early detection and treatment, my doctors forecast an eighty to eighty-five percent probability that all the cancer cells were killed.

I am your junior by a decade plus and re-entered college after working eight years. I have worked as a gas engineer and project manager for the past thirteen years. While working I visited local schools encouraging students to achieve in math and science and I served on the San Francisco Math Engineering Science Achievement Industrial Board for ten years. Two of those years I served as chairman and while chair I established a computer science laboratory for Math Engineering Science Achievement students. I share your commitment to educate our youth and I am available to support your efforts.

Another passion we share, is our love of Volvos and good rum. I have owned three and my favorite was the 122S I had while in college. I replaced just about every major component (engine, transmission and rear end) on the car to keep it running. I managed to save a bottle of Appleton Estate Extra from our last trip to Jamaica. We would love to share it with you on your next trip to the Bay Area. Please call us at (510 430-1215).

I read your book during my fifth week of treatment and it provided great mental relief during that painful period. Colin, I documenting my experiences to help me heal. Hopefully, the book will assist others seek regular medical exams and help people quick smoking. Attached for your review and recommendations is an overview of my book, Living Above The Line, A Family's Victory Over Cancer.

Colin, your support in the form of a letter of introduction to potential publisher(s) would be greatly appreciated.

Thanks

Gerald
Attachment

Living Above The Line, A Family's Victory Over Cancer chronicles a young African American male thirst for education through the troubled sixties. It covers the irony that a linear accelerator, a machine I reported on in the ninth grade (1964), would save my life thirty-one years later. The book tells of a love affair, the desire of a family to participate in the American Dream and work on potential solutions to help our country heal.

The cancer presented opportunities to redirect energies from career to healing and forced our family to explore alternative scenarios of achieving happiness and prosperity.

Please see brief description of book sections and list of potential chapters.

Section I
Consist of 3 chapters and provides some basic background on me from the sixth grade through high school.

Future Scientist
Chapter 1 The Mid Sixties
Chapter 2 Linear Accelerator Report
Chapter 3 Medicine In The South

Section II
Consist of 4 chapters and reviews life styles and options. This section will include statistical information on living standards for different segments of society.

Living Above The Line
Chapter 4 The Line
Chapter 5 The Road To The Line
Chapter 6 Make Your Choice
Chapter 7 Living With Your Choice

Section III
Consist of 3 chapters and reviews how I discovered I had cancer and reviews action plans.

The Discovery
Chapter 8 Found Out I Had Cancer
Chapter 9 Immediate Impact
Chapter 10 Identifying A Course Of Action

Section IV
Consist of 3 chapters and discusses the role of the various doctors and their impact on family life.

The Dream Team
Chapter 11 Review Doctors Roles
Chapter 12 Doctor Relationships
Chapter 13 Impact on life

Section V
Consist 4 chapters and chronicles my cancer treatment through life after treatment.

The Road To Recovery
Chapter 13 Implant Therapy
Chapter 14 External Radiation Treatment
Chapter 15 The Beat Goes On
Chapter 16 Pushing The Positive

General Colin L. Powell, USA (Retired)
Suite 767
909 North Washington Street
Alexandria, Virginia 22314

2 Dec

Dear Mr. Green,

Thanks for your note. I hope your recovery is complete. Appleton and Volvos will help!

Because of a large volume of similar requests, I can't help with a publisher's introduction. But best of luck,

C.P.

Monica
By Gerald Green

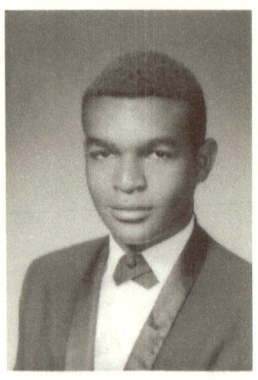

Gerald's
Cancer Discovered
Emotions Explored
Life Constricted
Love Tested

Gerald's
Pain Gathered
Softness Found
Life Constricted
Love Rediscovered

Gerald's
Radiation Delivered
Tumors Killed
Life Constricted
Love Flowed

Gerald's
Skin Burned
Sores Healed
Life Constricted
Love Exhales
Monica

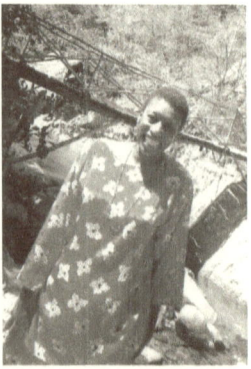